Other books in the Dx/Rx Series from Jones & Bartlett Learning

Dx/Rx:

Liver Cancer

Ghassan K. Abou-Alfa, MD
Gastrointestinal Service
Memorial Sloan-Kettering Cancer Center
Weill-Medical College
Cornell University
New York, New York

Celina Ang, MD
Fellow, Gastrointestinal Oncology
Memorial Sloan-Kettering Cancer Center
New York, New York

Series Editor: Manish A. Shah, MD
Director, Gastrointestinal Oncology Program
Division of Hematology and Medical Oncology
The Weill Cornell Solid Tumor Practice
New York, New York

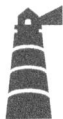

JONES & BARTLETT
LEARNING

World Headquarters
Jones & Bartlett Learning
5 Wall Street
Burlington, MA 01803
978-443-5000
info@jblearning.com
www.jblearning.com

Jones & Bartlett Learning books and products are available through most bookstores and online booksellers. To contact Jones & Bartlett Learning directly, call 800-832-0034, fax 978-443-8000, or visit our website, www.jblearning.com.

Substantial discounts on bulk quantities of Jones & Bartlett Learning publications are available to corporations, professional associations, and other qualified organizations. For details and specific discount information, contact the special sales department at Jones & Bartlett Learning via the above contact information or send an email to specialsales@jblearning.com.

Production Credits

Executive Publisher: Christopher Davis
Associate Editor: Laura Burns
Director of Production: Amy Rose
Senior Production Editor: Renée Sekerak
Marketing Manager: Rebecca Rockel
Manufacturing and Inventory Control
  Supervisor: Amy Bacus

Composition: Cenveo Publisher Services
Cover Design: Kate Ternullo
Cover Image: © CLIPAREA | Custom
  media ShutterStock, Inc.
Printing and Binding: Malloy, Inc.
Cover Printing: Malloy, Inc.

Library of Congress Cataloging-in-Publication Data
Abou-Alfa, Ghassan K.
  Dx/Rx. Liver cancer / Ghassan K. Abou-Alfa, Celina Ang.
    p. ; cm.
  Liver cancer
  Includes bibliographical references and index.
  ISBN 978-1-4496-4686-8 (pbk. : alk. paper)
  I. Ang, Celina. II. Title. III. Title: Liver cancer.
  [DNLM: 1. Liver Neoplasms—therapy—Handbooks. WI 39]

  616.99'436—dc23
                            2011035739

6048
Printed in the United States of America
15 14 13 12 11   10 9 8 7 6 5 4 3 2 1

Contents

Editor's Preface

Welcome to the Dx/Rx Oncology Series. The unique hand-books in this series provide important management and treatment information for the practicing physician in an easy-to-access bulleted format.

Dx/Rx: Liver Cancer is an exceedingly timely addition to the series, as the incidence of hepatocellular cancer (HCC) has increased and its management has become more and more complex. Drs. Abou-Alfa and Ang share their world-class expertise in the management of HCC in this thorough yet concise handbook describing the challenges of diagnosing and managing HCC in the context of underlying liver disease. This professional reference offers comprehensive coverage of fundamental topics in liver cancer, from the complexities of the different scoring systems of liver disease (ie, Childs-Pugh, MELD, and CUPI, among others) to the epidemiology and biology of HCC. Importantly, it includes a detailed outline of the local/regional, liver transplant, and systemic management options for HCC patients.

I am certain you will find this handbook to be an essential reference as you begin to manage these complex patients. As new drugs and treatment paradigms are developed for this disease, *Dx/Rx: Liver Cancer* will also serve as an invaluable resource for placing new therapies into context of current standards of care. I am sure you will enjoy this and other Dx/Rx Oncology editions, each of which is superb in its own right.

Manish A. Shah, MD

Introduction

The management of hepatocellular carcinoma (HCC) is challenging. HCC is a major source of morbidity and mortality worldwide. HCC is often referred to as "two diseases in one"; the clinician must consider not only the tumor, but also the underlying hepatic dysfunction that could promote tumorigenesis and significantly limit treatment options in patients with advanced disease. An understanding of the risk factors and geographic distribution associated with HCC can help to identify at-risk individuals who stand to benefit from surveillance and screening protocols. In those suspected to have HCC, investigations aimed at confirming the diagnosis, adequately mapping the extent and pattern of disease spread, and determining the degree of liver dysfunction are necessary steps in developing the optimal management plan.

Advances in surgical techniques and the judicious use of liver transplantation now provide a potentially curative option to patients who are diagnosed with HCC at an early enough stage to be amenable to such therapies. Percutaneous locoregional ablative therapies are options for patients who are diagnosed with early-stage disease but are not considered to be surgically resectable. Most importantly, patients with advanced, unresectable HCC—once considered an untreatable condition—now have therapeutic options in the form of targeted agents, which can control disease and prolong survival. Nevertheless, the quest to better understand how the biology of HCC interacts with these new agents remains a work in progress.

The purpose of this book is to provide the clinician caring for the patient with HCC with a practical resource outlining the risk factors, epidemiology, diagnosis, and management of this disease. In addition, it includes an overview of screening recommendations for at-risk patients, the molecular biology of HCC, and future areas of investigation in HCC research.

Ghassan K. Abou-Alfa, MD
Celina Ang, MD

Notice

We have made every attempt to summarize accurately and concisely a multitude of references. However, the reader is reminded that times and medical knowledge change, transcription or understanding error is always possible, and crucial details can be omitted whenever such a comprehensive distillation as this is attempted in a limited space. The primary purpose of this compilation is to cite literature on various sides of controversial issues; knowing where "truth" lies is usually difficult. We cannot, therefore, guarantee that every bit of information is absolutely accurate or complete. The reader should affirm that cited recommendations are reasonable by reading the original articles and checking other sources, including local consultants and recent literature, before applying them.

Drugs and medical devices are discussed that may have limited availability controlled by the Food and Drug Administration (FDA) for use only in research study or clinical trial. The drug information presented has been derived from reference sources, recently published data, and pharmaceutical tests. Research, clinical practice, and government regulations often change the accepted standard in this field. When consideration is being given to the use of any drug in the clinical setting, the clinician or reader is responsible for determining FDA status of the drug, reading the package insert, and prescribing information for the most up-to-date recommendations on dose, precautions, and contraindications and determining the appropriate usage for the product. This is especially important in the case of drugs that are new or seldom used.

CHAPTER 1

Epidemiology

■ Epidemiology of Hepatocellular Carcinoma (HCC)

- Hepatocellular carcinoma (HCC) ranks third among the main causes of worldwide cancer mortality behind lung and gastric cancer.[1]
  - The mortality rate is almost equivalent to the incidence rate (598,000 versus 626,000 yearly).
    - In 2002, over 80% of cases occurred in sub-Saharan Africa, eastern and southeastern Asia, and Melanesia. The incidence of HCC in China alone was 55%.
      - In China, the high prevalence of chronic hepatitis B virus (HBV) infection (up to 75% in Asia-Pacific countries excluding Japan)[2] has been held responsible for the high burden of HCC. Consumption of contaminated drinking water and betel quid in some parts of China, as will be discussed later, are other well-known risk factors.
      - Infection with HBV is also a major etiologic factor in Africa, where approximately 18% of the world's HBV carriers reside. Transmission occurs both vertically and horizontally, with local behavioral, cultural, and environmental practices playing a possible role.[3,4]
      - In Egypt, HCC is increasing exponentially as a leading cause of cancer morbidity and mortality. HCC represented 45% of all newly diagnosed gastrointestinal cancers between 2001

and 2002, and mortality has quadrupled since 1981.[5] Up to 14% of the Egyptian population is infected with hepatitis C virus (HCV), the highest rate worldwide.[6] This is partly due to a national treatment program against schistosomiasis, another known risk factor for HCC, in which the use of nondisposable needles potentially served as a conduit for transmission.[7,8]

- Low incidence areas include North America, most of Europe, Australia and New Zealand, parts of the Middle East, Latin America, and south central Asia (2.6–6.2 cases/100,000).[1]
  - The male:female incidence ratio is 2.4.[1]
- In the United States, HCC is the ninth leading cause of cancer mortality.
  - According to the American Cancer Society and the Surveillance, Epidemiology and End Results (SEER) database, 26,190 new diagnoses of primary liver cancers and intrahepatic cholangiocarcinomas and 19,590 deaths due to these diseases are expected to occur in 2011.[9]
- A recent review of the epidemiology of HCC in the United States revealed the following trends[10]:
  - Incidence and mortality rates increased the most among black, Hispanic, and white men age 50–59 years. Asians/Pacific Islanders had the highest incidence rates overall at 10–12%.
  - The 2- and 4-year survival rates doubled between 1992 and 2004 and were attributed to improved screening procedures and treatment options.
- The fibrolamellar variant of HCC (FLL-HCC) is a distinct diagnostic entity with unique clinical and treatment implications.
  - FLL-HCC is an extremely rare disease comprising < 1% of all primary liver cancers diagnosed. However, the prevalence might actually be higher given that some tumors may be misdiagnosed as typical HCC.
  - FLL-HCC occurs equally in younger individuals (in the third or fourth decade of life) of both sexes without

underlying liver disease. It also tends to occur more frequently in whites.[11]

■ Risk Factors

Hepatocarcinogenesis typically begins with an acute or chronic insult that induces liver remodeling with resulting fibrosis and cirrhosis. Age, sex, racial/ethnic, and geographic differences also modulate individual susceptibilities to developing HCC.

- Viral hepatitis
  - HBV and HCV are the leading risk factors for HCC, accounting for 75% of cases worldwide and 85% of cases in developing countries.[1] Infection with either of these viruses increases the risk of developing HCC by 20-fold.[12]
  - HCV predominates in Western populations, whereas HBV is more frequent in Asian populations.
  - Hepatocarcinogenesis due to HBV or HCV appears to arise by different mechanisms:
    - HBV DNA inserts into the host genome, disrupting key regulatory oncogenes by insertional mutagenesis. Chronic inflammation due to the host immune response may also destabilize the genome, permitting the accumulation of transforming mutations leading to HCC.[13,14]
    - The major mechanism of HCV hepatocarcinogenesis is thought to result from oxidative DNA damage and inflammation,[15] which gives rise to cirrhosis and, eventually, HCC in a process that spans 10–30 years. Viral proteins can also modulate host immune responses and intracellular signaling pathways, resulting in malignant transformation.[16] Iron overload states, chronic alcohol use, and metabolic syndrome can exacerbate HCV-induced damage.[17–19]
    - HBV carcinogenesis can occur in the absence of liver cirrhosis, whereas HCV-infected patients tend to develop HCC in the presence of cirrhosis.

- The incidence of HCC in HBV carriers is highest in those who are actively replicating, as indicated by the presence of envelope antigens and high levels of HBV DNA.[20,21] Although antiviral therapy can significantly decrease the risk of progression to HCC,[22] the risk remains elevated in chronic inactive carriers and following the clearance of surface antigens.[23,24]
    - An important consideration in chronic HBV carriers undergoing anticancer therapy for HCC is the potential for reactivation with deleterious clinical outcomes. This issue will be discussed further in Chapter 7: Management.
- Maintenance low-dose pegylated interferon does not decrease the risk of hepatocellular carcinogenesis in chronic HCV carriers who did not respond to ribavirin or pegylated interferon.[25]
- Alcohol
    - Excessive alcohol consumption is a well-recognized risk factor for HCC. Hepatocarcinogenesis results from the directly hepatotoxic effects of alcohol and the development of alcoholic cirrhosis.[26]
    - Alcohol-induced liver damage occurs through several mechanisms:
        - Alcohol dehydrogenase metabolizes alcohol into acetaldehyde, which decreases cell growth, causes apoptosis, and interferes with DNA synthesis.[27]
        - Alcohol induces cytochrome P450 enzyme 2E1, which converts a number of procarcinogens into carcinogens such as nitrosamines, aflatoxins, benzenes, and vinyl chloride.[28]
        - Alcohol induces free radical formation, which depletes antioxidants.[29] This causes lipid peroxidation, which is damaging to DNA and has been shown to disrupt p53 tumor suppressor activity.[30]
        - Folate, vitamin B_6, and vitamin B_{12} deficiencies due to malnutrition decrease antioxidant production and interfere with DNA methylation, which, in turn, may cause gene dysregulation and hepatocarcinogenesis.[29]
        - Chronic alcohol use may also be immunosuppressive.[31]

- Heavy alcohol consumption can potentiate liver damage caused by viral hepatitis and diabetes,[18] as well as smoking[32] and aflatoxins.[33]
  - The powerful synergy of alcohol with viral hepatitis and diabetes was illustrated in a case-control study conducted at MD Anderson Cancer Center. The odds ratios for the risk of developing HCC were 15.3, 12.6, 4.5, and 4.3 for the presence of anti-HCV antibodies, HBV surface antigens, heavy alcohol consumption, and diabetes mellitus, respectively. When the effect of alcohol was added to chronic viral hepatitis infection and diabetes, the odds ratios rose to 53.9 and 9.9, respectively.[18]
- Tobacco
  - Data on smoking as a risk factor for HCC have been inconsistent. Although some investigators have found that smoking-induced hepatotoxicity can lead to HCC,[34] several series from Europe, Asia, and South Africa have found no association.[35–37]

Metabolic Disorders

- Metabolic syndrome
  - Obesity, diabetes mellitus, and nonalcoholic steatohepatitis (NASH) are all independent risk factors for hepatocarcinogenesis.[19,38,39]
  - The metabolic syndrome is associated with peripheral insulin resistance and upregulation of the insulin/insulin-like growth factor-1 receptor (IGF-1R), a known mitogen that has been implicated in the development of multiple cancers.[40]
  - NASH also leads to HCC through the development of cryptogenic or idiopathic cirrhosis.[41]
- Hereditary hemochromatosis (HH)
  - HH is characterized by iron overload resulting from dysfunction of the iron-sensing apparatus.[42]
    - HH is caused by mutations of the *HFE* gene in association with decreased expression of hepcidin, a key protein involved in iron homeostasis.[42,43] The C282Y polymorphism is responsible for the

vast majority of cases; 90% of affected patients of Northern European descent are homozygotes.[44]

- ■ The H63D polymorphism is found in the general population and has variable penetrance.[45]
- • Untreated iron overload leads to hepatic fibrosis, cirrhosis, and diabetes mellitus.[46]
- • Iron overload also promotes the generation of free radicals, potentiating oxidative damage caused by alcohol and fibrosis due to viral hepatitis.[47]
- • Excess ferritin can also be immunosuppressive.[48]
- • Patients with HH have a 20- to 220-fold higher risk of HCC, but the risk does not appear to be elevated among first-degree relatives.[49,50]
- • Early phlebotomy may prevent or even reverse fibrosis and cirrhosis, thereby decreasing the risk of developing HCC.[49,51] However, HCC can also occur in the absence of iron overload and cirrhosis in these patients.[52]
- • The *HFE* gene mutation may also increase the susceptibility of patients with a history of viral hepatitis or excessive alcohol consumption to developing HCC.[53]
- ■ Alpha-1-antitrypsin (AAT) deficiency
  - • AAT is a serine protease inhibitor found in hepatocytes. AAT deficiency is an autosomal dominant inherited condition manifested by pulmonary emphysema, necrotizing panniculitis, cirrhosis, and HCC, as well as several multisystem autoimmune disorders.[54]
  - • Liver injury results from the accumulation of AAT glycoprotein in the endoplasmic reticulum of hepatocytes.[55]
  - • AAT-deficient patients with and without cirrhosis can develop HCC, possibly as a result of the carcinogenic effects of intracellular AAT accumulation. Cholangiocarcinomas and mixed hepatocholangiocarcinomas have also been observed among *PiZ* heterozygotes.[56]

Environmental Toxins

- ■ Aflatoxin
  - • Aflatoxins are produced by the *Aspergillus* fungus, which contaminates corn, peanuts, and grain products.[57,58,59]

- High consumption rates correlate with geographic high HCC incidence areas such as sub-Saharan Africa, Thailand, and Egypt.[60]
- Carcinogenesis occurs as a result of p53 tumor suppressor mutations due to the transversion of G → T at codon 249.[61,62] Like alcohol, aflatoxin exposure can potentiate the toxicity of viral hepatitis infections.[63]
- Betel quid chewing
  - Betel quid consumption is a popular practice in several Asian countries. The major carcinogenic ingredient in betel quid is the arecoline alkaloid.[64] Areca nuts grow on Areca palms, which are found in tropical regions.[65]
  - Mouse models have shown that toxicity occurs through several mechanisms.[64]
    - Arecoline causes immunosuppression by inducing splenic lymphocyte DNA damage, cell cycle arrest, and apoptosis in a dose-dependent manner.
    - Structural hepatocyte injury is manifested by the distortion of normal organelle architecture, cytoplasmic vacuoles, and decreased nuclear size and content. These changes are associated with elevations in transaminases.
    - Antioxidants, including superoxide dismutase and catalase, are suppressed.
  - The hepatotoxic effects of betel quid chewing have also been shown to be synergistic with HBV or HCV infection.[66]
  - As with alcohol and tobacco, betel nut consumption has also been implicated in cancers of the aerodigestive tract, including esophageal and squamous cell head and neck cancers.[67,68]
- Contaminated drinking water
  - The consumption of pond and ditch water contaminated with microcystins, a blue-green algal hepatotoxin, has been linked with a higher incidence of HCC in parts of rural China.[69,70]
  - There are several mechanisms of microcystin-associated hepatotoxicity, including:

- Inhibition of protein phosphatases, resulting in increased protein kinase activation, changes in hepatocyte morphology, and hepatotoxicity.[71]
- Oxidative DNA damage with concurrent decreases in free radical scavenging molecules such as glutathione.[72]
- Induction of apoptosis by increasing expression of p53 and Bax while suppressing expression of the antiapoptotic protein Bcl-2.[73]
- Co-exposure to aflatoxins and microcystins, which increases the risk of HCC in mouse models compared to exposure to either factor on its own. Exposure to aflatoxins and microcystins in the presence of the HBV x gene may further enhance the risk of hepatocarcinogenesis over time.[74]

Sex Differences

- HCC occurs 1.5 to 11 times more frequently in men than in women.[1]
- The differential effects of androgens and estrogens on hepatocytes provide a biological basis for the sex disparity.[75]
  - Androgens enhance the carcinogenicity of toxins like nitrosamines, and HBV X proteins (HBx) can activate androgen receptor transcriptional activity, also promoting carcinogenesis.[76,77]
  - In contrast, estrogens appear to exert a protective effect by suppressing Kupffer cell secretion of the proinflammatory cytokines.[78] Knockout or downregulation of the estrogen receptor-α by hypermethylation or microRNA miR-18a overexpression can lead to hepatocarcinogenesis.[79,80]
- Polymorphisms of the androgen receptor in men and women have been shown to interact with the HBV virus and modulate the risk of developing HCC.[81,82]

■ Protective Factors

- Coffee
  - Coffee consumption appears to be inversely related to the risk of developing HCC.[83,84] The antioxidants in

coffee appear to be responsible for many of its beneficial effects.

- Among individuals with risk factors for HCC, coffee and caffeine consumption has been associated with decreased levels of transaminases as markers of hepatocellular injury.[85,86]
- Coffee drinkers also have a lower risk of developing cirrhosis, and coffee may help to mitigate hepatotoxicity due to smoking.[87]

■ References

1. Parkin DM, Bray F, Ferlay J, et al. Global cancer statistics. *CA Cancer J Clin* 2005;55:74–108.
2. Yuen MF, Hou JL, Chutaputti A. Hepatocellular carcinoma in the Asia pacific region. *J Gastroenterol Hepatol* 2009;24:346–353.
3. Kramvis A, Kew MC. Epidemiology of hepatitis B virus in Africa, its genotypes and clinical associations of genotypes. *Hepatol Res* 2007;37(Suppl 1):S9–S19.
4. McClune AC, Tong MJ. Chronic hepatitis B and hepatocellular carcinoma. *Clin Liver Dis* 2010;14:461–476.
5. Elattar I. Magnitude of liver cancer in Egypt. October 2003. National Cancer Institute of Egypt. Available at: http://www.nci.edu.eg/lectures/cancer_problem/Magnitude%20of%20problem%20liver%20Cancer.pdf. Accessed December 15, 2010.
6. Lehman EM, Wilson ML. Epidemiology of hepatitis viruses among hepatocellular carcinoma cases and healthy people in Egypt: a systematic review and meta-analysis. *Int J Cancer* 2009;124:690–697.
7. Frank C, Mohamed MK, Strickland GT, et al. The role of parenteral antischistosomal therapy in the spread of hepatitis C virus in Egypt. *Lancet* 2000;355:887–891.
8. Strickland GT. Liver disease in Egypt: hepatitis C superseded schistosomiasis as a result of iatrogenic and biological factors. *Hepatology* 2006;43:915–922.
9. Siegel R, Ward E, Brawley O, et al. Cancer statistics, 2011: the impact of eliminating socioeconomic and racial disparities on premature cancer deaths. *CA Cancer J Clin* 2011;61(4):212–236.
10. Altekruse SF, McGlynn KA, Reichman ME. Hepatocellular carcinoma incidence, mortality, and survival trends in the United States from 1975 to 2005. *J Clin Oncol* 2009;27:1485–1491.

11. El-Serag HB, Davila JA. Is fibrolamellar carcinoma different from hepatocellular carcinoma? A US population-based study. *Hepatology* 2004;39:798–803.

12. Donato F, Boffetta P, Puoti M. A meta-analysis of epidemiological studies on the combined effect of hepatitis B and C virus infections in causing hepatocellular carcinoma. *Int J Cancer* 1998;75:347–354.

13. Cougot D, Neuveut C, Buendia MA. HBV induced carcinogenesis. *J Clin Virol* 2005;34(Suppl 1):S75–S78.

14. Lupberger J, Hildt E. Hepatitis B virus-induced oncogenesis. *World J Gastroenterol* 2007;13:74–81.

15. Maki A, Kono H, Gupta M, et al. Predictive power of biomarkers of oxidative stress and inflammation in patients with hepatitis C virus-associated hepatocellular carcinoma. *Ann Surg Oncol* 2007;14:1182–1190.

16. Tsai WL, Chung RT. Viral hepatocarcinogenesis. *Oncogene* 2010;29:2309–2324.

17. Furutani T, Hino K, Okuda M, et al. Hepatic iron overload induces hepatocellular carcinoma in transgenic mice expressing the hepatitis C virus polyprotein. *Gastroenterology* 2006;130:2087–2098.

18. Hassan MM, Huang LY, Hatten CJ, et al. Risk factors for hepatocellular carcinoma: synergism of alcohol with viral hepatitis and diabetes mellitus. *Hepatology* 2002;36:1206–1213.

19. Ohki T, Tateishi R, Sato T, et al. Obesity is an independent risk factor for hepatocellular carcinoma development in chronic hepatitis C patients. *Clin Gastroenterol Hepatol* 2008;6:459–464.

20. Yang HI, Lu SN, Liaw YF, et al. Hepatitis B e antigen and the risk of hepatocellular carcinoma. *N Engl J Med* 2002; 347:168–174.

21. Chen CJ, Yang HI, Su J, et al. Risk of hepatocellular carcinoma across a biological gradient of serum hepatitis B virus DNA level. *JAMA* 2006;295:65–73.

22. Sung JJ, Tsoi KK, Wong VW, et al. Meta-analysis: treatment of hepatitis B infection reduces the risk of hepatocellular carcinoma. *Aliment Pharmacol Ther* 2008;28:1067–1077.

23. Chen JD, Yang HI, Illoeje UH, et al. Carriers of inactive hepatitis B virus are still at risk for hepatocellular carcinoma and liver-related death. *Gastroenterology* 2010;138:1747–1754.

24. Simonetti J, Bulkow L, McMahon BJ, et al. Clearance of hepatitis B surface antigen and risk of hepatocellular carcinoma in a cohort chronically infected with hepatitis B virus. *Hepatology* 2010;51:1531–1537.

25. Lok AS, Seeff LB, Morgan TR, et al. Incidence of hepatocellular carcinoma and associated risk factors in hepatitis C-related advanced liver disease. *Gastroenterology* 2009;136: 138–148.

26. Lieber CS. Alcohol and the liver: 1994 update. *Gastroenterology* 1994;106:1085–1105.
27. Clemens DL, Forman A, Jerrells TR, et al. Relationship between acetaldehyde levels and cell survival in ethanol-metabolizing hepatoma cells. *Hepatology* 2002;35:1196–1204.
28. Anderson LM, Chhabra SK, Nerurkar PV, et al. Alcohol-related cancer risk: a toxicokinetic hypothesis. *Alcohol* 1995;12:97–104.
29. Voigt MD. Alcohol in hepatocellular cancer. *Clin Liver Dis* 2005;9:151–169.
30. Hu H, Feng Z, Eveleigh J, et al. The major lipid peroxidation product, trans-4-hydroxy-2-nonenal, preferentially forms DNA adducts at codon 249 of human p53 gene, a unique mutational hotspot in hepatocellular carcinoma. *Carcinogenesis* 2002;23:1781–1789.
31. Roselle G, Mendenhall CL, Grossmann C. Effects of alcohol on immunity and cancer. In: Yirmiya R, Taylor AN (eds). *Alcohol, Immunity and Cancer*. Boca Raton, FL: CRC Press, 1993:3–22.
32. Kuper H, Tzonou A, Kaklamani E, et al. Tobacco smoking, alcohol consumption and their interaction in the causation of hepatocellular carcinoma. *Int J Cancer* 2000;85:498–502.
33. Bulatao-Jayme J, Almero EM, Castro CA. A case–control dietary study of primary liver cancer risk from aflatoxin exposure. *Int J Epidemiol* 1982;11:112–119.
34. El-Zayadi AR. Heavy smoking and liver. *World J Gastroenterol* 2006;12:6098–6101.
35. Mayans MV, Calvet X, Bruix J, et al. Risk factors for hepatocellular carcinoma in Catalonia, Spain. *Int J Cancer* 1990;46:378–381.
36. Tanaka K, Hirohata T, Takashita S, et al. Hepatitis B virus, cigarette smoking and alcohol consumption in the development of hepatocellular carcinoma: a case-control study in Fukuoka, Japan. *Int J Cancer* 1992;51:509–514.
37. Mohamed AE, Kew C, Groeneveld HT. Alcohol consumption as a risk factor for hepatocellular carcinoma in urban southern African blacks. *Int J Cancer* 1992;51:537–541.
38. Pagano G, Pacini G, Musso G, et al. Nonalcoholic steatohepatitis, insulin resistance, and metabolic syndrome: further evidence for an etiologic association. *Hepatology* 2002;35:367–372.
39. Starley BQ, Calcagno CJ, Harrison SA. Nonalcoholic fatty liver disease and hepatocellular carcinoma: a weighty connection. *Hepatology* 2010;51:1820–1832.
40. Fair AM, Montgomery K. Energy balance, physical activity and cancer risk. *Methods Mol Biol* 2009;472:57–88.
41. Bugianesi E. Non-alcoholic steatohepatitis and cancer. *Clin Liver Dis* 2007;11:191–207.

42. Pietrangelo A. Hereditary hemochromatosis: pathogenesis, diagnosis, and treatment. *Gastroenterology* 2010;139:393–408.
43. Feder JN, Gnirke A, Thomas W, et al. A novel MHC class I-like gene is mutated in patients with hereditary haemochromatosis. *Nat Genet* 1996;13:399–408.
44. Merryweather-Clarke AT, Pointon JJ, Shearman JD, et al. Global prevalence of putative haemochromatosis mutations. *J Med Genet* 1997;34:275–278.
45. Gochee PA, Powell LW, Cullen DJ, et al. A population-based study of the biochemical and clinical expression of the H63D hemochromatosis mutation. *Gastroenterology* 2002;122:646–651.
46. Adams PC, Duegnier Y, Moirand R, et al. The relationship between iron overload, clinical symptoms, and age in 410 patients with genetic hemochromatosis. *Hepatology* 1997; 25:162–166.
47. Hultcrantz R, Bissell DM, Roll FJ. Iron mediates production of a neutrophil chemoattractant by rat hepatocytes metabolizing ethanol. *J Clin Invest* 1991;87:45–49.
48. Bacon BR, Britton RS. The pathology of hepatic iron overload: a free radical-mediated process? *Hepatology* 1990;11:127–137.
49. Niederau C, Fischer R, Sonnenberg A, et al. Survival and causes of death in cirrhotic and non-cirrhotic patients with primary hemochromatosis. *N Engl J Med* 1985; 313:1256–1262.
50. Elmberg M, Hultcrantz R, Ekbom A, et al. Cancer risk in patients with hereditary hemochromatosis and in their first-degree relatives. *Gastroenterology* 2003;125:1733–1741.
51. Blumberg RS, Chopra S, Ibrahim R, et al. Primary hepatocellular carcinoma in idiopathic hemochromatosis after reversal of cirrhosis. *Gastroenterology* 1988;95:1399–1402.
52. Singh P, Kaur H, Lerner RG, et al. Hepatocellular carcinoma in non-cirrhotic liver without evidence of iron overload in a patient with primary hemochromatosis. Review. *J Gastrointest Cancer* [Epub ahead of print on September 28, 2010]
53. Fargion S, Stazi MA, Fracanzani AL, et al. Mutations in the HFE gene and their interaction with exogenous risk factors in hepatocellular carcinoma. *Blood Cells Mol Dis* 2001;27:505–511.
54. Silverman EK, Sandhaus RA. Clinical practice. Alpha-1-antitrypsin deficiency *N Engl J Med* 2009;360:2749–2757.
55. Fairbanks KD, Tavill AS. Liver disease in alpha-1-antitrypsin deficiency: a review. *Am J Gastroenterol* 2008;103:2136–2141.
56. Zhou H, Fischer HP. Liver carcinoma in PiZ alpha-1-antitrypsin deficiency. *Am J Surg Pathol* 1998;22:742–748.
57. Anand R. Aflatoxins. In: *IARC Monograph on the Evaluation of Carcinogenic Risks to Humans. Vol. 82. Some Traditional*

Herbal Medicines Some Mycotoxins, Naphthalene and Styrene. New York: McGraw-Hill, 2002:171–300.

58. Cornell University, Department of Animal Science. Aflatoxins: occurrence and health risk. March 26, 2009. Available at: http://www.ansci.cornell.edu/plants/toxicagents/aflatoxin/aflatoxin.html. Accessed January 5, 2011.

59. Queensland Government, Primary Industries and Fisheries. Aflatoxin in peanuts. October 13, 2010. Available at: http://www.dpi.qld.gov.au/26_11899.htm. Accessed January 5, 2011.

60. Van Rensburg SJ, Cook-Mozaffari P, Van Schalkwyk DJ, et al. Hepatocellular carcinoma and dietary aflatoxin in Mozambique and Trantskei. *Br J Cancer* 1985;51:713–726.

61. Bressac B, Kew M, Wands J, et al. Selective G to T mutations of p53 in hepatocellular carcinoma from southern Africa. *Nature* 1991;350:429–431.

62. Hsu IC, Metcalf RA, Sun T, et al. Mutational hotspot in the p53 gene in human hepatocellular carcinomas. *Nature* 1991;350:427–428.

63. Ghebranious N, Sell S. Hepatitis B injury, male gender, aflatoxin, and p53 expression each contribute to hepatocarcinogenesis in transgenic mice. *Hepatology* 1998;27:383–391.

64. Dasgupta R, Saha I, Pal S, et al. Immunosuppression, hepatotoxicity and depression of antioxidant status by arecoline in albino mice. *Toxicology* 2006;227:94–104.

65. India Development Gateway, Agriculture. Areca nut. January 12, 2009. Available at: http://www.indg.in/agriculture/crop_production_techniques/areca-nut. Accessed January 5, 2011.

66. Tsai JF, Chuang LY, Jeng JE, et al. Betel quid chewing as a risk factor for hepatocellular carcinoma: a case-control study. *Br J Cancer* 2001;84:709–713.

67. Pickwell SM, Schimelpfening S, Palinkas LA, et al. "Betelmania." Betel quid chewing by Cambodian women in the United States and its potential health effects. *West J Med* 1994;160:326–330.

68. Goldenberg D, Lee J, Koch WM, et al. Habitual risk factors for head and neck cancer. *Otolaryngol Head Neck Surg* 2004;131:986–993.

69. Ueno Y, Nagata S, Tsutsumi T, et al. Detection of microcystins, a blue-green algal hepatotoxin, in drinking water sampled in Haimen and Fusui, endemic areas of primary liver cancer in China, by highly sensitive immunoassay. *Carcinogenesis* 1996;17:1317–1321.

70. Yu SZ. Primary prevention of hepatocellular carcinoma. *J Gastroenterol Hepatol* 1995;10:674–682.

71. Carmichael WW, Azevedo SM, An JS, et al. Human fatalities from cyanobacteria: chemical and biological evidence for cyanotoxins. *Environ Health Perspect* 2001;109:663–668.

72. Zegura B, Lah TT, Filipic M. Alteration of intracellular GSH levels and its role in microcystin-LR-induced DNA damage in human hepatoma HepG2 cells. *Mutat Res* 2006;611:25–33.

73. Fu WY, Chen JP, Wang XM, et al. Altered expression of p53, Bcl-2 and Bax induced by microcystin-LR in vivo and in vitro. *Toxicon* 2005;46:171–177.

74. Lian M, Liu Y, Yu XZ, et al. Hepatitis B virus x gene and cyano-bacterial toxins promote aflatoxin B1-induced hepatotumori-genesis in mice. *World J Gastroenterol* 2006;12:3065–3072.

75. Yeh SH, Chen PJ. Gender disparity of hepatocellular carcinoma: the roles of sex hormones. *Oncology* 2010;78(Suppl 1):172–179.

76. Ma WL, Hsu CL, Wu MH, et al. Androgen receptor is a new potential therapeutic target for the treatment of hepa-tocellular carcinoma. *Gastroenterology* 2008;135:947–955.

77. Chiu CM, Yeh SH, Chen PJ, et al. Hepatitis B virus X pro-tein enhances androgen receptor-responsive gene expres-sion depending on androgen level. *Proc Natl Acad Sci USA* 2007;104:2571–2578.

78. Naugler WE, Sakurai T, Kim S, et al. Gender disparity in liver cancer due to sex differences in MyD88-dependent IL-6 production. *Science* 2007;317:121–124.

79. Shen L, Ahuja N, Shen Y, et al. DNA methylation and en-vironmental exposures in human hepatocellular carcinoma. *J Natl Cancer Inst* 2002;94:755–761.

80. Liu WH, Yeh SH, Lu CC, et al. MicroRNA-18a prevents estrogen receptor-alpha expression, promoting prolifera-tion of hepatocellular carcinoma cells. *Gastroenterology* 2009;136:683–693.

81. Yu MW, Cheng SW, Lin MW, et al. Androgen-receptor gene CAG repeats, plasma testosterone levels, and risk of hepatitis B-related hepatocellular carcinoma. *J Natl Cancer Inst* 2000;92:2023–2028.

82. Yu MW, Yang YC, Yang SY, et al. Androgen receptor exon 1 CAG repeat length and risk of hepatocellular carcinoma in women. *Hepatology* 2002;36:156–163.

83. Bravi F, Bosetti C, Tavani A, et al. Coffee consumption and hepatocellular carcinoma risk: a meta-analysis. *Hepatology* 2007;46:430–435.

84. Larsson SC, Wolk A. Coffee consumption and risk of liver can-cer: a meta-analysis. *Gastroenterology* 2007;132:1740–1745.

85. Ruhl CE, Everhart JE. Coffee and caffeine consumption re-duce the risk of elevated serum alanine aminotransferase ac-tivity in the United States. *Gastroenterology* 2005;128:24–32.

86. Casiglia E, Spolaore P, Ginocchio G, et al. Unexpected effects of coffee consumption on liver enzymes. *Eur J Epidemiol* 1993;9:293–297.

87. Klatsky AL, Armstrong MA. Alcohol, smoking, coffee, and cirrhosis. *Am J Epidemiol* 1992;136:1248–1257.

Clinical Features

■ Presenting Signs and Symptoms

▦ There are no clinical signs or symptoms that are pathognomonic of hepatocellular carcinoma (HCC).

▦ Patients may present with systemic symptoms such as malaise, fatigue, anorexia, and weight loss.

▦ Abdominal discomfort due to hepatomegaly and/or a liver mass, capsular stretching, and inflammation may be present.

▦ Acute abdominal pain and distension due to the spontaneous rupture of a superficial tumor with resulting hemoperitoneum is a common presentation of HCC in high-incidence regions, although it is less common in Western populations (≤ 5%).[1] It usually occurs in patients with underlying cirrhosis, although exceptions have been reported.[2] This potentially fatal event is a medical emergency that warrants early recognition and management.

  ● Tumor rupture with hemoperitoneum can be diagnosed with high certainty on contrast-enhanced computed tomography scans. Hemoperitoneum appears as hyperdense intraperitoneal fluid. Contrast extravasation from the ruptured wall of a peripheral or subcapsular lesion is often seen[1] (**Figure 2.1**). Emergent surgery or local therapy may be indicated for patients with preserved liver function or those with advanced cirrhosis, respectively.[1–3]

▦ Right upper quadrant pain, jaundice, and hyperbilirubinemia are indicative of biliary obstruction.

▦ Some patients may have stigmata of chronic liver disease including palmar erythema, clubbing, leukonychia, spider angiomata, ascites, and caput medusae (periumbilical

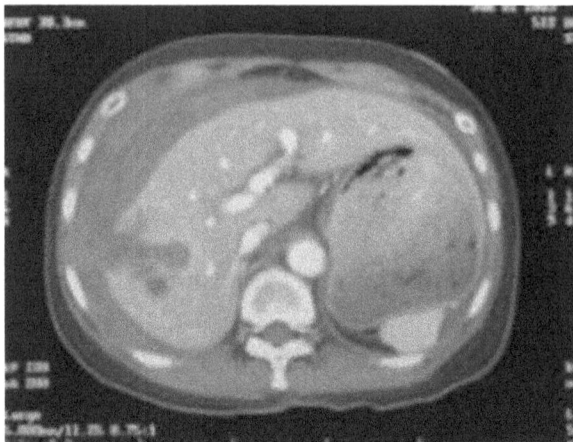

Figure 2.1   Tumor Rupture with Hemoperitoneum

venous dilation). In those with compensated cirrhosis, acute hepatic decompensation (variceal bleed, encephalopathy, jaundice) may herald the development of HCC.

- Although a fever must initiate a workup for an infectious cause, it may also reflect the release of inflammatory mediators such as cytokines and tumor necrosis.

■ Laboratory Tests

- Laboratory results tend to be nonspecific and often reflect underlying liver dysfunction.
- Hyperbilirubinemia and elevations in liver transaminases, alkaline phosphatase, and γ-glutamyltransferase are often seen.
- Hepatic synthetic dysfunction may be reflected by low albumin levels and abnormal coagulation indices.
  - The international normalized ratio (INR) reflects hepatic synthesis of fibrinogen and vitamin K–dependent coagulation factors. It is often normal in patients with early or mild cirrhosis. Changes in the INR can occur quickly because some clotting factors have a short half-life, but a persistent increase indicates progressive liver dysfunction and failure.[4]

- The INR has been optimized for monitoring patients on warfarin, but may not always accurately reflect the degree of coagulopathy due to hepatic dysfunction depending on the kind of assay reagents used.[5,6] This can impact the Model for End-Stage Liver Disease (MELD) scores of transplant candidates, thereby influencing patient prioritization and organ allocation.[6]
  - Prothrombin time does not accurately reflect coagulopathy in cirrhotic patients.[7]
- Hypoalbuminemia occurs in patients with advanced cirrhosis due to decreased synthesis of albumin (reflected by levels < 30 g/dL) as well as dilution from hypervolemia. The half-life of albumin is approximately 3 weeks, so there is a delay between the onset of decreased synthesis and detectable laboratory abnormalities.[4]
- Patients may have anemia due to chronic disease.
- Blood urea nitrogen and creatinine may become elevated due to hepatorenal syndrome caused by tumor and/or hepatic decompensation. Mild electrolyte abnormalities may also be present.
  - Hepatorenal syndrome occurs when portal hypertension causes splanchnic vasodilation, leading to a drop in mean arterial pressure and renal hypoperfusion. In response to this perceived intravascular hypovolemia, activation of the renin-angiotensin and sympathetic nervous systems and secretion of antidiuretic hormone (ADH) cause renal vasoconstriction and increased salt and water retention, resulting in edema, hyponatremia, and worsening renal failure.[8]

■ Paraneoplastic Syndromes

HCC can be associated with several metabolic derangements. The presence of paraneoplastic syndromes is an independent poor prognosticator. In one series, patients survived a median of only 36 days following the clinical detection of a paraneoplastic syndrome.[9]

- Hypertension
  - Case reports have described tumor production of compounds involved in the renin-angiotensin-aldosterone

system, causing arterial hypertension in previously normotensive patients.[10–12] For example, gene polymorphisms of angiotensinogen (AGT), a compound produced by hepatocytes, are involved in the pathogenesis of essential hypertension.[13] AGT-producing HCC tumors have been reported.[12]

- Hypoglycemia
  - Tumor-associated hypermetabolism and the production of insulin agonists like insulin-like growth factor-2 (IGF-2) increase glucose consumption, causing hypoglycemia.[14,15]
  - IGF-2 and other markers of the insulin/insulin-like growth factor axis have been implicated in hepatocarcinogenesis,[16,17] and targeted therapies against this pathway have been developed and are currently being evaluated in clinical trials.

- Erythrocytosis
  - Serum erythropoietin (EPO) levels have been found to be elevated in patients with HCC but are not consistently associated with erythrocytosis. Patients with erythrocytosis may have normal serum EPO levels.[18]
  - Erythrocytosis may occur in response to hypoxic stress or may result from autonomous EPO production by HCC cells.[19] Immunohistochemical studies have demonstrated cytoplasmic EPO in HCC tumor cells but not in surrounding normal hepatocytes.[20] The expression of mutant forms of EPO mRNA has been documented in HCC tumors.[21]
  - Patients with erythrocytosis appear to survive longer than those with other paraneoplastic syndromes.[9]

- Hypercalcemia
  - Hypercalcemia may result from osteolytic metastases or reflect hypercalcemia of malignancy as a result of parathyroid hormone-related peptide (PTHrP) secretion by tumor cells.[22,23]

- Hypercholesterolemia
  - Paraneoplastic hypercholesterolemia has been reported in 15–25% of patients with HCC.[24,25]
  - The mechanism underlying paraneoplastic hypercholesterolemia may result from the decreased expression

of low-density lipoprotein (LDL) receptors by HCC cells, resulting in decreased LDL cholesterol clearance. This may be associated with loss of heterozygosity of chromosome 19p13.2.[26] In addition, rat models suggest that aberrant expression of genes controlling cholesterol efflux and homeostasis as well as decreased bile acid synthesis may be contributory.[27]

Although erythrocytosis and hypercholesterolemia appear to be earlier paraneoplastic manifestations of HCC, hypercalcemia and hypoglycemia are considered to be harbingers of end-stage disease.[9]

- Diarrhea
  - Markers of neuroendocrine differentiation have been reported in HCC[28] and have provided the basis for treating HCC with somatostatin analogs, albeit with variable success.[29,30] The release of neuroendocrine hormones such as vasoactive intestinal peptide and 5-hydroxytryptamine has also been documented in patients with diarrhea later found to have HCC.[31]
  - Diarrhea also appears to be more frequent among cirrhotic patients who develop HCC than those who do not.[32]
- Gynecomastia
  - Gynecomastia has been reported as a presenting symptom in male patients with fibrolamellar HCC (FLL-HCC) in association with tumor aromatase overexpression.[33–35]

■ Paraneoplastic Dermatoses Associated with HCC

Several dermatologic conditions have been found to be associated with gastrointestinal malignancies including HCC.[36,37] These include the following:

- Dermatomyositis
  - Findings include myalgias and muscle weakness. The classic dermatologic signs are Gottron's papules (scaly, erythematous lesions on the extensor surfaces of the metacarpals, interphalangeal joints, elbows, and knees), the shawl sign (V-shaped erythematous rash involving the shoulders, upper back, and chest), and a violaceous, heliotropic rash of the upper eyelids.[37,38]

- The sign of Leser-Trélat refers to eruptive seborrheic keratoses, which are sharply demarcated, scaly, hyperpigmented lesions with a "stuck on" appearance.[37]
- Pemphigus
  - Paraneoplastic pemphigus is an autoimmune blistering disorder involving the skin and mucus membranes. Although it is most often associated with lymphoproliferative disorders, there are case reports of it occurring with solid tumors, including HCC.[39]
  - Pemphigus foliaceus is similar to paraneoplastic pemphigus except that it does not involve the mucus membranes. It, too, has been reported in a patient with HCC in conjunction with acanthosis nigricans.[40]
- Pityriasis rotunda
  - Pityriasis rotunda is characterized by sharply demarcated, round or oval, scaly patches usually found on the trunk, buttocks, or extremities.[41]
  - The prevalence of pityriasis rotunda is significantly higher in South African blacks with HCC than in matched controls and may be a marker of HCC in this population.[42]
- Porphyria cutanea tarda (PCT)
  - Decreases in the activity of uroporphyrinogen decarboxylase, an enzyme involved in heme biosynthesis, lead to uroporphyrinogen accumulation in the blood and urine.[43]
  - Cutaneous manifestations include a photosensitivity rash characterized by hyperpigmentation, hirsutism, and vesicobullae formation, which may become hemorrhagic.[44]
  - PCT has been associated with hepatitis C virus infection and is a risk factor for the development of HCC.[45]

■ Patterns of Metastatic Spread

- Up to 20% of patients have distant metastases at diagnosis or recurrence.
- The likelihood of having distant metastases is related to tumor size and gross histologic subtype; tumors > 5 cm in diameter have a significantly higher frequency of intra- and extrahepatic metastases.[46]

- The regional and abdominal lymph nodes, lungs, bones, peritoneum, and adrenals are common sites of extrahepatic metastases.[46–48]
- Bone metastases may be facilitated by increased circulating levels of vascular endothelial growth factor (VEGF); serum VEGF levels were found to be significantly higher in patients with HCC bone metastases than those without. Primary and bone metastases also demonstrated immunoreactivity for VEGF.[49]
- The development of extrahepatic metastases represents more advanced disease and portends a worse prognosis.[48,50]

■ References

1. Castells L, Moreiras M, Quiroga S, et al. Hemoperitoneum as a first manifestation of hepatocellular carcinoma in western patients with liver cirrhosis: effectiveness of emergency treatment with transcatheter arterial embolization. *Dig Dis Sci* 2001;46:555–562.
2. Abdel Samie A, Otto G, Thielmann L. Acute hemoperitoneum due to spontaneous tumor rupture as first manifestation of hepatocellular carcinoma. *Z Gastroenterol* 2007;45: 615–619.
3. Recodare A, Bonariol L, Caratozzolo E, et al. Management of spontaneous bleeding due to hepatocellular carcinoma. *Minerva Chir* 2002;57:347–356.
4. Shaffer EA. Testing for hepatic and biliary disorders. Laboratory tests. Merck Manual Online. June 2009. Available at: http://www.merckmanuals.com/professional/sec03/ch023/ch023b.html. Accessed December 20, 2010.
5. Deitcher SR. Interpretation of the international normalized ratio in patients with liver disease. *Lancet* 2002;359:47–48.
6. Trotter JF, Brimhall B, Arjal R, et al. Specific laboratory methodologies achieve higher model for endstage liver disease (MELD) scores for patients listed for liver transplantation. *Liver Transpl* 2004;10:995–1000.
7. Tripodi A, Salerno F, Chantarangkul V, et al. Evidence of normal thrombin generation in cirrhosis despite abnormal conventional coagulation tests. *Hepatology* 2005;41:553–558.
8. Gines P, Schrier RW. Renal failure in cirrhosis. *N Engl J Med* 2009;361:1279–1290.
9. Luo JC, Hwang SJ, Wu JC, et al. Clinical characteristics and prognosis of hepatocellular carcinoma patients with paraneoplastic syndromes. *Hepatogastroenterology* 2002;49: 1315–1319.

10. Arai H, Saitoh H, Matsumoto T, et al. Hypertension as a paraneoplastic syndrome in hepatocellular carcinoma. *J Gastroenterol* 1999;34:530–534.

11. Kew MC, Leckie BJ, Greeff MC, et al. Arterial hypertension as a paraneoplastic phenomenon in hepatocellular carcinoma. *Arch Intern Med* 1989;149:2111–2113.

12. Arai H, Saitoh S, Matsumoto T, et al. Hypertension as a paraneoplastic syndrome in hepatocellular carcinoma. *J Gastroenterol* 1999;34:530–534.

13. Jeunemaitre X, Soubrier F, Kotelevtsev YV, et al. Molecular basis of human hypertension. Role of angiotensinogen. *Cell* 1992;71:169–180.

14. Tietge UJ, Schofl C, Ocran KW, et al. Hepatoma with severe non-islet cell tumor hypoglycemia. *Am J Gastroenterol* 1998;93:997–1000.

15. Eastman RC, Carson RE, Orloff DG, et al. Glucose utilization in a patient with hepatoma and hypoglycemia. Assessment by a positron emission tomography. *J Clin Invest* 1992;89:1958–1963.

16. Desbois-Mouthon C, Baron A, Blivet-Van Eggelpoël MJ, et al. Insulin-like growth factor-1 receptor inhibition induces a resistance mechanism via the epidermal growth factor receptor/HER3/AKT signaling pathway: rational basis for co-targeting insulin-like growth factor-1 receptor and epidermal growth factor receptor in hepatocellular carcinoma. *Clin Cancer Res* 2009;15:5445–5456.

17. Feitelson MA, Pan J, Lian Z. Early molecular and genetic determinants of primary liver malignancy. *Surg Clin North Am* 2004;84:339–354.

18. Kew MC, Fisher JW. Serum erythropoietin concentrations in patients with hepatocellular carcinoma. *Cancer* 1986;58:2485–2488.

19. Matsuyama M, Yamazaki O, Horii K, et al. Erythrocytosis caused by an erythropoietin-producing hepatocellular carcinoma. *J Surg Oncol* 2000;75:197–202.

20. Sakisaka S, Watanabe M, Tateishi H, et al. Erythropoietin production in hepatocellular carcinoma cells associated with polycythemia: immunohistochemical evidence. *Hepatology* 1993;18:1357–1362.

21. Funakoshi A, Muta H, Baba T, et al. Gene expression of mutant erythropoietin in hepatocellular carcinoma. *Biochem Biophys Res Commun* 1993;195:717–722.

22. Knill-Jones RP, Buckle RM, Parsons V, et al. Hypercalcemia and increased parathyroid-hormone activity in a primary hepatoma. Studies before and after hepatic transplantation. *N Engl J Med* 1970;282:704–708.

23. Yen TC, Hwang SJ, Wang CC, et al. Hypercalcemia and parathyroid hormone-related protein in hepatocellular carcinoma. *Liver* 1993;13:311–315.

24. Hwang SJ, Lee SD, Chang CF, et al. Hypercholesterolaemia in patients with hepatocellular carcinoma. *J Gastroenterol Hepatol* 1992;7:491–496.

25. Ndububa DA, Ojo OS, Adetiloye VA, et al. The incidence and characteristics of some paraneoplastic syndromes of hepatocellular carcinoma in Nigerian patients. *Eur J Gastroenterol Hepatol* 1999;11:1401–1404.

26. Sohda T, Iwata K, Kitamura Y, et al. Reduced expression of low-density lipoprotein receptor in hepatocellular carcinoma with paraneoplastic hypercholesterolemia. *J Gastroenterol Hepatol* 2008;23:e153–e156.

27. Hirayama T, Honda A, Matsuzaki Y, et al. Hypercholesterolemia in rats with hepatomas: increased oxysterols accelerate efflux but do not inhibit biosynthesis of cholesterol. *Hepatology* 2006; 44:602–611.

28. Zhao M, Laissue JA, Zimmermann A. "Neuroendocrine" differentiation in hepatocellular carcinomas (HCCs): immunohistochemical reactivity is related to distinct tumor cell types, but not to tumor grade. *Histol Histopathol* 1993;8:617–626.

29. Guo TK, Hao XY, Ma B, et al. Octreotide for advanced hepatocellular carcinoma: a meta-analysis of randomized controlled trials. *J Cancer Res Clin Oncol* 2009;135:1685–1692.

30. Jia WD, Zhang CH, Xu GL, et al. Octreotide therapy for hepatocellular carcinoma: a systematic review of the evidence from randomized controlled trials. *Hepatogastroenterology* 2010;57:292–299.

31. Giannelli G, Pierri F, Schiraldi O, et al. Diarrhea as first clinical manifestation of hepatocellular carcinoma. *Recenti Prog Med* 2002;93:478–481.

32. Bruix J, Castells A, Calvet X, et al. Diarrhea as a presenting symptom of hepatocellular carcinoma. *Dig Dis Sci* 1990; 35:681–685.

33. Agarwal VR, Takayama K, Van Wyk JJ, et al. Molecular basis of severe gynecomastia associated with aromatase expression in a fibrolamellar hepatocellular carcinoma. *Clin Endocrinol Metab* 1998;83:1797–1800.

34. Hany MA, Betts DR, Schmugge M, et al. A childhood fibrolamellar hepatocellular carcinoma with increased aromatase activity and a near triploid karyotype. *Med Pediatr Oncol* 1997;28:136–138.

35. McCloskey JJ, Germain-Lee EL, Perman JA, et al. Gynecomastia as a presenting sign of fibrolamellar carcinoma of the liver. *Pediatrics* 1988;82:379–382.

36. Gregory B, Ho VC. Cutaneous manifestations of gastrointestinal disorders. Part II. *J Am Acad Dermatol* 1992;26: 371–383.

37. Thiers BH, Sahn RE, Callen JP. Cutaneous manifestations of internal malignancy. *CA Cancer J Clin* 2009;59:73–98.

38. Mammen AL. Dermatomyositis and polymyositis: clinical presentation, autoantibodies and pathogenesis. *Ann NY Acad Sci* 2010;1184:134–153.

39. Hinterhuber G, Drach J, Riedl E, et al. Paraneoplastic pemphigus in association with hepatocellular carcinoma. *J Am Acad Dermatol* 2003;49:538–540.

40. Muramatsu T, Matsumoto H, Yamashina Y, et al. Pemphigus foliaceus associated with acanthosis nigricans-like lesions and hepatocellular carcinoma. *Int J Dermatol* 1989;28: 462–463.

41. Rao J, Metelitsa A, Lin A, et al. Pityriasis rotunda. Available at: http://emedicine.medscape.com/article/1107624-overview. Accessed November 28, 2010.

42. Berkowitz I, Hodkinson HJ, Kew MC, et al. Pityriasis rotunda as a cutaneous marker of hepatocellular carcinoma: a comparison with its prevalence in other diseases. *Br J Dermatol* 1989;120:545–549.

43. Kushner JP, Barbuto AJ, Lee GR. An inherited enzymatic defect in porphyria cutanea tarda: decreased uroporphyrinogen decarboxylase activity. *J Clin Invest* 1976;58:1089–1097.

44. Cripps DJ. Diet and alcohol effects on the manifestation of hepatic porphyrias. *Fed Proc* 1987;46:1894–1900.

45. Lim HW, Mascaro JM. The porphyrias and hepatocellular carcinoma. *Dermatol Clin* 1995;13:135–142.

46. Yuki K, Hirohashi S, Sakamoto M, et al. Growth and spread of hepatocellular carcinoma. A review of 240 consecutive autopsy cases. *Cancer* 1990;66:2174–2179.

47. Otebagyo JA, Atalabi OM, Yakubu A. Clinicoradiologic and sonographic patterns of metastasis in hepatocellular carcinoma. *J Natl Med Assoc* 2006;98:1620–1622.

48. Tonolini M, Solbiati L, Ierace T, et al. Extrahepatic recurrence and second malignancies after treatment of hepatocellular carcinoma: spectrum of imaging findings. *Radiol Med (Torino)* 2002;103:196–205.

49. Iguchi H, Uchimura K, Yokota M, et al. Increased incidence of bone metastases and its management in hepatocellular carcinoma (HCC) [abstract]. *Proc Am Soc Clin Oncol* 2003; 22:1250.

50. Yang Y, Nagano H, Ota H, et al. Patterns and clinicopathologic features of extrahepatic recurrence of hepatocellular carcinoma after curative resection. *Surgery* 2007;141: 196–202.

Diagnostic Workup

■ Introduction

Key elements of the diagnostic workup of hepatocellular carcinoma (HCC) include imaging, pathologic confirmation of the diagnosis, tumor markers, and liver function tests. These investigations provide important information about the cancer itself and underlying liver reserve, both of which, as will be discussed in subsequent chapters, influence treatment and prognosis.

■ Biopsy

A correct pathologic diagnosis is the cornerstone of oncologic management; tumor staging and subsequent therapy are determined by this key diagnostic step. However, better imaging modalities as well as an improved knowledge of the pathogenesis and natural history of HCC have encouraged several groups to question the need to biopsy all at-risk patients.

The Case Against Obtaining a Biopsy

- Several noninvasive diagnostic guidelines have been developed to help identify patients who may not require a biopsy to diagnose HCC. These are based on the size of the lesion, its enhancement characteristics on imaging, and serum α-fetoprotein (AFP) levels.
- The American Association for the Study of Liver Diseases (AASLD) diagnostic algorithm guides the workup of patients with known risk factors for HCC who are found to have a suspicious nodule on a screening ultrasound (see **Figure 3.1**).[1]

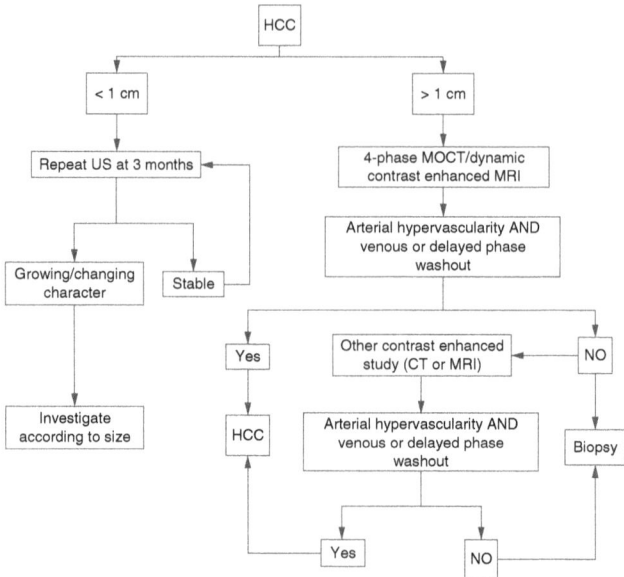

Figure 3.1 American Association for the Study of Liver Diseases Algorithm for the Workup of a Suspicious Liver Nodule

CT, computed tomography; MDCT, multidetector computed tomography; MRI, magnetic resonance imaging; US, ultrasound.

Source: This material is reproduced with permission of the American Association for the Study of Liver Diseases, www.aasld.org/Practice Guidelines, Management of hepatocellular carcinoma: an update. Alexandria, VA: American Association for the Study of Liver Diseases, 2010.

- Lesions < 1 cm are followed every 3–6 months for up to 2 years, and if they remain unchanged, the usual screening interval is resumed.
- Patients with lesions > 1 cm in diameter should undergo dynamic contrast-enhanced imaging with either a 4-phase multidetector computed tomography (CT) scan, or an magnetic resonance imaging (MRI).
- A diagnosis of HCC is made if the typical pattern of arterial enhancement followed by venous phase washout is observed. If not, a biopsy is indicated.

- The European Association for the Study of the Liver (EASL) noninvasive diagnostic criteria for HCC in patients with cirrhosis[2,3]:
  - Two imaging studies showing a hypervascular lesion > 2 cm in diameter *or*
  - One imaging study showing a hypervascular lesion > 2 cm in diameter *and* an AFP > 400 ng/mL
- The United Network for Organ Sharing (UNOS) organizes organ allocation. A biopsy is not mandatory for HCC patients being considered for transplantation, as long as it meets the following diagnostic imaging criteria[4]:
  - Abdominal CT or MRI to document the extent of disease, and a chest CT ruling out pulmonary metastases
  - The presence of a hepatic tumor ≥ 2 cm in diameter with one or more of the following: AFP > 200 ng/mL, "vascular blush," an arteriogram confirming the tumor, prior liver ablation or chemoembolization[3,4]
- Geographic and ethnic differences in the presentation and natural history of HCC may limit the applicability of guidelines developed for Western patients to an Asian patient population. In 2003, tailored recommendations were developed by the Korean Liver Cancer Study Group (KLCSG) and the National Cancer Center (NCC) for the diagnosis and management of HCC in Korean patients.[5]

The Case for Obtaining a Biopsy

- A major limitation of noninvasive diagnostic guidelines is their heavy reliance on imaging modalities that have limited sensitivity for small lesions. This is a critical consideration given that early detection of HCC provides the best chance for cure and better long-term outcomes.
  - Even the best imaging modalities currently available have limited diagnostic precision for lesions < 2 cm in diameter, particularly in cirrhotic livers.[6]
  - Although MRI has been shown to be better than CT, ultrasound, and serum AFP at diagnosing HCC in cirrhotic livers, its sensitivity and specificity are 80–85%.[7]

- Smaller lesions often have a nonspecific pattern and may mimic the appearance of regenerative or dysplastic nodules, which are common in cirrhotic livers.[6,8]
- Another pitfall of making a diagnosis of HCC based on imaging alone is the risk of false-positive results. Patients have been unnecessarily subjected to morbid therapies, including liver transplantation, as a result of being falsely diagnosed.
  - In one retrospective series, the false-positive rate was 20–33%, resulting in a significant increase in the rate of inappropriate organ allocations, particularly after the Model for End-Stage Liver Disease (MELD) scoring system was implemented (see Chapter 4).[9]
  - Up to 20% of patients nationally were found to have been misdiagnosed as having HCC following liver transplantation.[10]
  - The positive predictive value of helical CT and MRI, at best, ranges from approximately 60–70%.[11,12]
- Pathologic examination of tissue specimens allows for an assessment of tumor grade and differentiation, which gives insight into the underlying biology. Furthermore, specimens provide material for correlative biomarker studies that may help us to better understand the disease process, predict responses to therapy, and estimate prognosis. Recent clinical trials of targeted agents in HCC have identified several biomarkers associated with clinical outcomes, such as pERK with sorafenib[13] and circulating stem cells and inflammatory mediators with sunitinib.[14]
- A CT- or ultrasound-guided core biopsy is the optimal technique because it provides information on tumor architecture relative to normal liver parenchyma. As with any procedure, risks and benefits of biopsy must be weighed. There is a small but real risk of needle tract seeding (2.7% according to a meta-analysis), which must be considered, especially for patients being considered for potentially curative therapy.[15] Nevertheless, the importance of making an accurate diagnosis takes precedence, given its implications for management.

▨ Given the limitations of modern imaging techniques, biopsy of suspicious lesions and careful pathologic examination provide the most certainty for making the diagnosis of HCC and should be done in all patients who would be eligible for therapy. This is extremely important for ensuring that patients are managed appropriately for both the type and stage of disease. A biopsy may be forfeited in patients with severe liver dysfunction (e.g., Child-Pugh C cirrhosis), comorbidities, and/or a poor performance status for whom systemic therapy would not be justified.

▨ Imaging

Imaging of HCC is a continuously evolving science. Each of the following modalities presented has its limitations, and multiple factors influence the decision on which technique to use.

Computed Tomography (CT)

▨ A triphasic CT scan captures the hepatic arterial, portal venous, and delayed phases of contrast transit through the liver and is a commonly used modality for the radiologic diagnosis of HCC. Tumors typically hyperenhance on the arterial phase and then washout during the venous phase. The delayed phase captures isoattenuating lesions that would otherwise have been missed on a dual-phase CT.[16]

▨ Triphasic CT scans have high diagnostic accuracy, with a sensitivity and specificity of 89% and 99%, respectively.[16]

▨ In addition to their diagnostic utility and accessibility, triphasic CT scans may have a role in evaluating responses to antiangiogenic therapies.

• Significant increases in the ratio of tumor necrosis to tumor volume from baseline have been observed in patients responding to sorafenib.[13,17] (See **Figure 3.2.**)

▨ Multislice helical CTs are capable of faster and more detailed image acquisition, which is particularly advantageous during the finite period of contrast transit.[18,19]

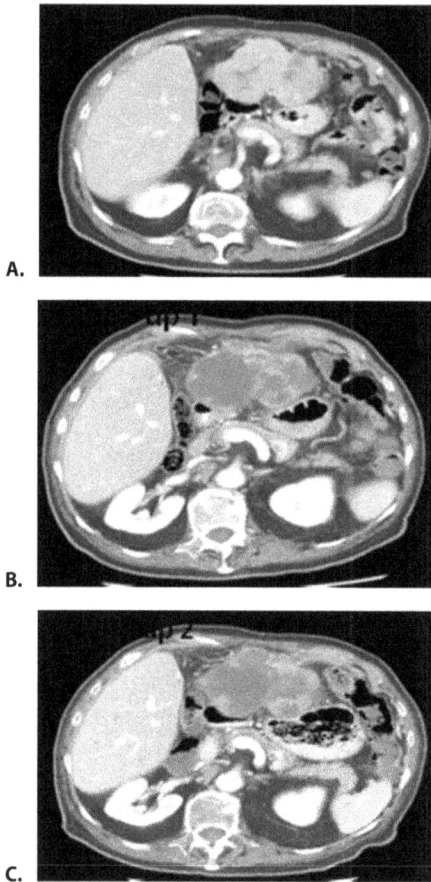

Figure 3.2   Tumor Necrosis

A. Baseline. **B.** Follow-up at 2 months. **C.** Follow-up at 4 months.

- Multidetector row helical CTs provide even greater diagnostic precision by capturing early and late arterial phase images.[20]
- False positives with helical CT scans have been reported in 8% of patients. Causes of false positives include dysplastic or regenerative nodules, fibrosis, fat, peliosis hepatis, and hemangiomas.[21]

Magnetic Resonance Imaging (MRI)

▪ Gadolinium-enhanced MRI is an accurate imaging modality for HCC. Compared to regular contrast-enhanced CT scans, MRI has the advantages of improved resolution, lack of ionizing radiation, and better sensitivity and specificity for the detection of premalignant lesions in cirrhotic patients; however, MRI is more expensive than CT.[11,22]

▪ Multiphase dynamic contrast-enhanced MRI (DCE-MRI) is analogous to a triphasic CT scan. In patients with cirrhosis, the sensitivity of this modality for detecting lesions > 2 cm in diameter is as high as 100%, but this drops significantly to 50% for lesions 1–2 cm and to 4% for lesions < 1 cm.[23]

▪ Features on MRI that suggest HCC are tumor size > 2 cm, T2 hyperintensity, T1 hypointensity, the presence of a fibrous capsule, and rapid growth.[24] The finding of delayed washout after arterial enhancement on DCE-MRI has been shown to predict the diagnosis of HCC in lesions < 2 cm with a sensitivity and specificity of 80% and 95%, respectively.[25]

▪ DCE-MRI may also have a role in response assessment to antiangiogenic therapies.

  ● Decreases in arterial enhancement and tumor vascularity have been correlated with responses to bevacizumab[26] and sunitinib,[27] respectively, but not sorafenib and doxorubicin.[28]

  ● Tumor necrosis on DCE-MRI has also been significantly correlated with pathologic confirmation of tumor necrosis following transarterial chemoembolization.[29] Given that tumor necrosis appears to correlate with patient outcomes on sorafenib,[13,17] this might be another potential application for DCE-MRI.

▪ Hepatic-specific contrast agents such as gabodenate dimeglunine (MultiHance by Bracco) and gadoxetate disodium (Eovist or Primovist by Bayer Healthcare) are currently used in clinical practice. These agents can differentiate hepatic tumors based on patterns of uptake by normal hepatocytes and biliary clearance.[30]

▪ Superparamagnetic iron oxide (SPIO) is a liver-specific contrast agent that is selectively taken up by phagocytic Kupffer cells, which are often absent from malignant tumors.[31] SPIO-enhanced MRI can therefore discriminate benign from malignant tumors[31] and has demonstrated high sensitivity for detecting small HCC tumors in cirrhotic livers.[32,33]

- Other new MRI contrast agents and imaging techniques are being developed that have the potential to provide information on tumor differentiation, vascularity, and oxygenation.[34–36] These advances, although promising, are not yet ready for routine clinical practice.

- CT or magnetic resonance arteriography can improve tumor detection and delineate tumor vascular anatomy as part of the preoperative evaluation. However, these techniques are invasive (contrast is injected into the superior mesenteric, splenic, or hepatic artery), are not widely available, and have not been shown to be more accurate than MRI.[37]

- The choice between using CT or MRI as the primary diagnostic imaging modality is ultimately dictated by local availability and expertise.

Ultrasonography (US)

- US is primarily used as a screening modality because it poorly discriminates between malignant and benign liver lesions, especially in cirrhotic livers.[38] HCC might be suspected on the basis of poorly defined margins and irregular, coarse echogenicity, but larger tumors become harder to distinguish from normal liver parenchyma.[39]

- Power or color Doppler US are useful for distinguishing between bland and malignant portal vein thrombosis.[38]

- Newer techniques that may broaden the clinical utility of US as a diagnostic tool have been developed.
  - Contrast-enhanced US (CEUS) diagnoses HCC based on enhancement characteristics during different vascular phases.[18] CEUS is also excellent for differentiating between malignant and bland portal venous thrombi.[40]
  - Tissue harmonic ultrasound uses the second harmonic frequencies generated by tissue reflection of the acoustic signal to create higher resolution images with less background noise, making it easier to distinguish cystic from solid masses.[41–43]

Positron Emission Tomography (PET)

▪ PET scans are not recommended for routine use in the diagnostic workup of HCC. Fluorodeoxyglucose (FDG) avidity appears to depend on tumor size and the degree of differentiation. Only 55–70% of HCCs are FDG avid, and these are often larger (> 5 cm), well-differentiated tumors.[44,45]

▪ PET might have better sensitivity for detecting distant pulmonary or bone metastases.[45]

▪ PET findings have a variable clinical significance. In one series, management was changed in 28% of cases based on PET results.[46]

■ Tumor Markers

Alpha-Fetoprotein (AFP)

▪ AFP is the universally accepted tumor marker for HCC. It is used to screen for and diagnose HCC, monitor response to therapy, and detect changes in disease burden.

▪ An AFP level > 500 µg/L in an at-risk patient is generally considered diagnostic of HCC.

▪ Several caveats limit the use of AFP alone in making the diagnosis of HCC, making it extremely important to consider the clinical context as well as other diagnostic investigations:

  ● AFP is not specific for HCC; elevations can be associated with pregnancy, gonadal tumors, and viral hepatitis.

  ● AFP may not be as reliable in early-stage HCC. In one series, up to 40% of patients with tumors ≤ 3 cm had a normal AFP, and some even had a spontaneous decrease from a previously elevated level.[47]

  ● The presence of an elevated AFP may depend on the etiology of underlying liver disease (viral hepatitis > alcoholic liver disease).[48] Also, the fibrolamellar subtype of HCC is frequently associated with a normal AFP.[49]

▪ AFP elevations due to cirrhosis versus HCC may be differentiated based on their associated sugar-chain structures.

  ● AFP *Lens culinaris* agglutinin A (AFP L3) and erythro-agglutinating phytohemagglutinin (AFP P4+P5) were found to be elevated only in patients with hepatitis B or C cirrhosis and HCC, and not those with cirrhosis alone. Furthermore, elevations in both forms of AFP predated the radiographic detection of HCC.[50] The use of these assays is still investigational.

Des-Gamma-Carboxyprothrombin (DCP)

- DCP is an abnormal form of prothrombin produced in association with vitamin K deficiency and/or liver dysfunction.[51]
- The degree of plasma DCP elevation was shown to differentiate HCC from normal patients and differentiate nonmalignant causes of liver disease and liver metastases from other primaries; it also appeared to correlate with disease activity. However, there was poor correlation between AFP and DCP.[52] The use of plasma DCP remains investigational.

Liver Function Tests

- Total and direct bilirubin, serum albumin, and the international normalized ratio (INR) are indices of synthetic liver function. Along with the clinical presence of ascites and/or encephalopathy, liver function tests are used to assign patients a Child-Pugh score, indicating the degree of hepatic dysfunction. This information has important implications for management and prognosis, as will be discussed in subsequent chapters.

Hepatitis B and C Viral Serology

- Infection with either hepatitis C virus (HCV) or hepatitis B virus (HBV) is a major risk factor for the development of HCC.
- Patients who are infected with HBV or HCV exhibit differential responses to systemic therapies like sorafenib; those with HCV cirrhosis appear to derive greater benefit.[52] This is believed to result from the upregulation of Raf1, a target of sorafenib, thereby improving tumor sensitivity to this drug.[53] Furthermore, sorafenib has been shown to block HCV replication in vitro.[54] This will be discussed in further detail in Chapter 7: Management.

■ References

1. Bruix J, Sherman M. AASLD Prace Guidelines. Management of hepatocellular carcinoma: an update. *Hepatology* July 2010. http://www.aasld.org/practiceguidelines/Documents/ Bookmarked%20Practice%20Guidelines/HCCUpdate2010.pdf.
2. Bruix J, Sherman M, Llovet JM, et al. Clinical management of hepatocellular carcinoma. Conclusions of the Barcelona-2000 EASL Conference. European Association for the Study of the Liver. *J Hepatol* 2001;35:421–430.
3. Bialecki ES, Azenekwe AM, Brunt AM, et al. Comparison of biopsy and non-invasive methods for diagnosis of hepatocellular carcinoma. *Clin Gastroenterol Hepatol* 2006;4:361–368.
4. Organ Procurement and Transplantation Network. 3.6 Allocation of livers. November 9, 2010. http://optn.transplant .hrsa .gov/PoliciesandBylaws2/policies/pdfs/policy_8.pdf.
5. Korean Liver Cancer Study Group and National Cancer Center. Practice guidelines for management of hepatocellular carcinoma 2009. *Korean J Hepatol* 2009;15:391–423.
6. Willatt JM, Hussain HK, Adusumilli S, et al. MR imaging of hepatocellular carcinoma in the cirrhotic liver: challenges and controversies. *Radiology* 2008;247:311–330.
7. Colli A, Fraquelli M, Casazza G, et al. Accuracy of ultrasonography, spiral CT, magnetic resonance, and alphafetoprotein in diagnosing hepatocellular carcinoma: a systematic review. *Am J Gastroenterol* 2006;101:513–523.
8. Baron RL, Peterson MS. Screening the cirrhotic liver for hepatocellular carcinoma with CT and MR imaging: opportunities and pitfalls. *Radiographics* 2001;21(Special Issue): S117–S132.
9. Hayashi PH, Trotter JF, Forman L, et al. Impact of pretransplant diagnosis of hepatocellular carcinoma on cadaveric liver allocation in the era of MELD. *Liver Transpl* 2004;10: 42–48.
10. Freeman RB, Harper A, Edwards E, et al. The MELD/ PELD system and hepatocellular carcinoma [abstract]. *Am J Transplant* 2003;3(Suppl 5):284.
11. Libbrecht L, Bielen D, Verslype C, et al. Focal lesions in cirrhotic explant livers: pathological evaluation and accuracy of pretransplantation imaging examinations. *Liver Transpl* 2002;8:749–761.
12. Brancatelli G, Baron RL, Peterson MS, et al. Helical CT screening for hepatocellular carcinoma in patients with cirrhosis: frequency and causes for false-positive interpretation. *AJR Am J Roentgenol* 2003;180:1007–1014.
13. Abou-Alfa GK, Schwartz L, Ricci S, et al. Phase II study of sorafenib in patients with advanced hepatocellular carcinoma. *J Clin Oncol* 2006;24:1–8.

14.   Zhu AX, Sahani DV, Duda DG, et al. Efficacy, safety, and potential biomarkers of sunitinib monotherapy in advanced hepatocellular carcinoma: a phase II study. *J Clin Oncol* 2009;27:3027–3035.

15.   Silva MA, Hegab B, Hyde C, et al. Needle track seeding following biopsy of liver lesions in the diagnosis of hepatocellular cancer: a systematic review and meta-analysis. *Gut* 2008;57:1592–1596.

16.   Lim JH, Choi D, Kim SH. Detection of hepatocellular carcinoma: value of adding delayed phase imaging to dual-phase helical CT. *AJR Am J Roentgenol* 2002;179:67–73.

17.   Abou-Alfa GK, Zhao B, Capanu M, et al. Tumor necrosis as a correlate for response in subgroup of patients with advanced hepatocellular carcinoma (HCC) treated with sorafenib. ESMO 2008, Stockholm, Sweden, Abstract 547P.

18.   Choi BI. The current status of imaging diagnosis of hepatocellular carcinoma. *Liver Transpl* 2004;10(2 Suppl 1): S20–S25.

19.   Hu H, He HD, Foley WD, et al. Four multidetector-row helical CT: image quality and volume coverage speed. *Radiology* 2000;215:55–62.

20.   Murakami T, Kim T, Takahashi S, et al. Hepatocellular carcinoma: multidetector row helical CT. *Abdom Imaging* 2002;27:139–146.

21.   Brancatelli G, Baron RL, Peterson MS, et al. Helical CT screening for hepatocellular carcinoma in patients with cirrhosis: frequency and causes of false-positive interpretation. *AJR Am J Roentgenol* 2003;180:1007–1014.

22.   Vauthey JN, Dixon E, Abdalla EK, et al. Pretreatment assessment of hepatocellular carcinoma: expert consensus statement. *HPB* 2010;12:289–299.

23.   Krinsky GA, Lee VS, Thiese ND, et al. Transplantation for hepatocellular carcinoma and cirrhosis: sensitivity of magnetic resonance imaging. *Liver Transpl* 2002;8:1156–1164.

24.   Ayyappan AP, Jhaveri KS. CT and MRI of hepatocellular carcinoma: an update. *Expert Rev Anticancer Ther* 2010;10: 507–519.

25.   Marrero JA, Hussain HK, Nghiem HV, et al. Improving the prediction of hepatocellular carcinoma in cirrhotic patients with an arterially-enhancing liver mass. *Liver Transpl* 2005;11:281–289.

26.   Siegel AB, Cohen EI, Ocean A, et al. Phase II trial evaluating the clinical and biologic effects of bevacizumab in unresectable hepatocellular carcinoma. *J Clin Oncol* 2008;26:2992–2998.

27.   Zhu AX, Sahani DV, Duda DG, et al. Efficacy, safety, and potential biomarkers of sunitinib monotherapy in advanced hepatocellular carcinoma: a phase II study. *J Clin Oncol* 2009;27:3027–3035.

28. Abou-Alfa GK, Gultekin DH, Capanu M, et al. Association of dynamic contrast enhanced-MRI (DCE-MRI) with response in a subgroup of patients with advanced hepatocellular carcinoma (HCC) treated with doxorubicin plus sorafenib. 2009 Gastrointestinal Cancers Symposium, San Francisco, CA, Abstract 271.

29. Mannelli L, Kim S, Hajdu C, et al. Assessment of tumor necrosis of hepatocellular carcinoma after chemoembolization: diffusion-weighted and contrast-enhanced MRI with histopathologic correlation of the explanted liver. *AJR Am J Roentgenol* 2009;193:1044–1052.

30. Fidler F, Hough D. Hepatocyte-specific magnetic resonance imaging contrast agents. *Hepatology* 2011;53:678–682.

31. Reimer P, Tombach B. Hepatic MRI with SPIO: detection and characterization of focal liver lesions. *Eur Radiol* 1998;8:1198–1204.

32. Kim YK, Kwak HS, Kim CS, et al. Hepatocellular carcinoma in patients with chronic liver disease: comparison of SPIO-enhanced MR imaging and 16–detector row CT. *Radiology* 2006;238:531–541.

33. Kim YK, Kim CS, Lee YH, et al. Comparison of superparamagnetic iron oxide-enhanced and gadobenate dimeglumine-enhanced dynamic MRI for detection of small hepatocellular carcinomas. *AJR Am J Roentgenol* 2004;182:1217–1223.

34. Vandecaveye V, De Keyzer F, Verslype C, et al. Diffusion-weighted MRI provides additional value to conventional dynamic contrast-enhanced MRI for detection of hepatocellular carcinoma. *Eur Radiol* 2009;19:2456–2466.

35. Catalano OA, Choy G, Zhu A, et al. Differentiation of malignant thrombus from bland thrombus of the portal vein in patients with hepatocellular carcinoma: application of diffusion-weighted MR imaging. *Radiology* 2010;254:154–162.

36. Naik M, Mannelli L, Chandarana H, et al. Hepatocellular carcinoma: assessment of tumor oxygenation with BOLD MRI. *Proc Intl Soc Mag Reson Med* 2008;16:3741.

37. Choi D, Kim S, Lim J, et al. Preoperative detection of hepatocellular carcinoma: ferumoxides-enhanced MR imaging versus combined helical CT during arterial portography and CT hepatic arteriography. *AJR Am J Roentgenol* 2001;176:475–482.

38. Bialecki ES, Bisceglie AM. Diagnosis of hepatocellular carcinoma. *HPB* 2005;7:26–34.

39. Ishiguchi T, Shimamoto K, Fukatsu H, et al. Radiologic diagnosis of hepatocellular carcinoma. *Semin Surg Oncol* 1996;12:164–169.

40. Tarantino L, Francica G, Sordelli I, et al. Diagnosis of benign and malignant portal vein thrombosis in cirrhotic patients with hepatocellular carcinoma: color Doppler US,

contrast-enhanced US, and fine-needle biopsy. *Abdom Imaging* 2006;31:537–544.

41.   Thomas JD, Rubin DN. Tissue harmonic imaging: why does it work? *J Am Soc Echocardiogr* 1998;11:803–808.

42.   Ward B, Baker AC, Humphrey VF. Nonlinear propagation applied to the improvement of resolution in diagnostic medical ultrasound. *J Acoust Soc Am* 1997;101:143–154.

43.   Tranquart F, Grenier N, Eder V, et al. Clinical use of ultrasound tissue harmonic imaging. *Ultrasound Med Biol* 1999;25:889–894.

44.   Wolfort RM, Papillion PW, Turnage RH, et al. Role of FDG-PET in the evaluation and staging of hepatocellular carcinoma with comparison of tumor size, AFP level, and histologic grade. *Int Surg* 2010;95:67–75.

45.   Khan MA, Combs CS, Brunt EM, et al. Positron emission tomography scanning in the evaluation of hepatocellular carcinoma. *J Hepatol* 2000;32:792–797.

46.   Wudel LJ, Delbeke D, Morris D, et al. The role of [18F]fluoro-deoxyglucose positron emission tomography imaging in the evaluation of hepatocellular carcinoma. *Am Surg* 2003;69:117–124.

47.   Chen DS, Sun JL, Sheu JC, et al. Serum alpha-fetoprotein in the early stage of human hepatocellular carcinoma. *Gastroenterology* 1984;86:1404–1409.

48.   Fasani P, Sangiovanni A, De Fazio C, et al. High prevalence of multinodular hepatocellular carcinoma in patients with cirrhosis attributable to multiple risk factors. *Hepatology* 1999;29:1704–1707.

49.   Stipa F, Yoon SS, Liau KH, et al. Outcome of patients with fibrolamellar hepatocellular carcinoma. *Cancer* 2006;106:1331–1338.

50.   Sato Y, Nakata K, Kato Y, et al. Early recognition of hepatocellular carcinoma based on altered profiles of alpha-fetoprotein. *N Engl J Med* 1993;328:1802–1806.

51.   Stenflo J, Suttie JW. Vitamin K-dependent formation of gamma-carboxyglutamic acid. *Annu Rev Biochem* 1977;46:157–172.

52.   Liebman HA, Furie BC, Tong MJ, et al. Des-gamma-carboxy (abnormal) prothrombin as a serum marker of primary hepatocellular carcinoma. *N Engl J Med* 1984;310:1427–1431.

53.   Huitzil FD, Saltz LS, Song J, et al. Retrospective analysis of outcome in hepatocellular carcinoma (HCC) patients (pts) with hepatitis C (C+) versus B (B+) treated with sorafenib (S). 2008 Gastrointestinal Cancers Symposium, January 19–21, 2008, Orlando, FL, Abstract 173.

54.   Giambartolomei S, Covone F, Levrero M, et al. Sustained activation of the Raf/MEK/Erk pathway in response to EGF in stable cell lines expressing the hepatitis C virus (HCV) core protein. *Oncogene* 2001;20:2606–2610.

55.   Himmelsbach K, Sauter D, Baumert TF, et al. New aspects of an anti-tumor drug: sorafenib efficiently inhibits HCV replication. *Gut* 2009;58:1644–1653.

CHAPTER 4

Staging and Prognosis

■ Introduction

Staging helps to classify the extent of disease, guide therapy, and provide prognostic information. While most cancers are staged according to anatomic parameters, in hepatocellular carcinoma (HCC), it has become apparent that the degree of underlying liver dysfunction also influences therapeutic options and impacts survival.[1,2] Numerous combined anatomic and functional staging systems have been proposed in an effort to incorporate these considerations.

■ Measures of Underlying Liver Dysfunction

The Child-Pugh classification scheme and Model for End-Stage Liver Disease (MELD) are established systems for risk stratification and prognostication in patients with cirrhosis.

Child-Pugh Classification (Table 4.1)

- Serum albumin, prothrombin time measured as the international normalized ratio (INR), bilirubin, and the presence of clinically apparent ascites and hepatic encephalopathy are used to group patients according to the degree of hepatic dysfunction.[3,4] The Child-Pugh score has been used to predict the risk of developing complications of cirrhosis, perioperative morbidity and mortality, and has been shown to correlate with survival.[5-7]
  - One- and 2-year survival rates for Child-Pugh classes are as follows: class A, 100% and 85%; class B, 80% and 60%; and class C, 45% and 35%, respectively.

Table 4.1   The Child-Pugh Scoring System for Liver Cirrhosis

	Points		
	1	2	3
Albumin	> 3.5 g/dL	2.8–3.5 g/dL	< 2.8 g/dL
Total bilirubin	< 2 mg/dL	2–3 mg/dL	> 3 mg/dL
INR	< 1.7	1.7–2.3	> 2.3
Clinical ascites	Absent	Mild	Moderate
Clinical encephalopathy	Absent	Grade 1–2	Grade 3–4

A = 5–6 points; B = 7–9 points; C ≥ 10 points.

- Its limitations include the subjectivity of grading the clinical parameters, the validity of equally weighting each variable, and the arbitrary cut-off levels established for each variable. Furthermore, other variables known to impact prognosis such as serum creatinine and the presence of portal vein thrombosis are not included.[8]

Model for End-Stage Liver Disease (MELD; Table 4.2)

- MELD is a more contemporary scoring system that was initially designed to predict short-term mortality in cirrhotic patients undergoing transhepatic intrahepatic portosystemic shunt (TIPS) procedures. Serum

Table 4.2   Estimated 3-Month Survival by Model for End-Stage Liver Disease (MELD) Score

MELD Score	3-Month Mortality
> 40	71.3%
30–39	52.6%
20–29	19.6%
10–19	6%
< 9	1.9%

INR, creatinine, and bilirubin levels are used to predict 3-month mortality in patients with end-stage cirrhosis who are being considered for liver transplantation.[9,10]

- MELD = 3.8 [Ln serum bilirubin (mg/dL)] + 11.2 (Ln INR) + 9.6 [Ln serum creatinine (mg/dL)] + 6.4.
- A MELD score calculator is available at http://www.mayoclinic.org/MELD.

■ Staging Systems

Anatomic Only: The American Joint Committee on Cancer (AJCC)/Union Internationale Contre le Cancer (UICC) Tumor, Node, Metastases (TNM) Systems

- The 2002 (sixth) edition of the AJCC/UICC TNM classification is the only staging system to have been validated as prognostic of outcome in patients who have undergone liver transplantation as primary treatment for HCC.[11] The seventh edition of the TNM system was published in 2010. This updated version created separate staging systems for HCC and intrahepatic cholangiocarcinoma, split the T3 category to reflect the different prognoses of large multifocal lesions versus the presence of macrovascular invasion, redefined the N1 category, and classified lymph node metastases as stage IV disease.[12] The seventh edition TNM categories and stage groupings are as follows.
- T stage categories
  - T0 – no detectable tumor
  - T1 – solitary lesion without vascular invasion
  - T2 – solitary lesion with vascular invasion *or* multiple lesions each ≤ 5 cm in diameter
  - T3a – multiple lesions > 5 cm in diameter
  - T3b – tumor(s) of any size invading a main branch of the portal or hepatic vein
  - T4 – tumor(s) directly invades adjacent organs (aside from gallbladder) or perforates the visceral peritoneum
- N stage categories
  - N0 – no regional lymph node involvement
  - N1 – regional lymph node involvement (includes inferior phrenic nodes)

- M stage categories
  - M0 – no distant metastases
  - M1 – distant metastases present
- Stage groupings
  - Stage I – T1N0M0
  - Stage II – T2N0M0
  - Stage IIIA – T3aN0M0
  - Stage IIIB – T3bN0M0
  - Stage IIIC – T4N0M0
  - Stage IVA – $T_{any}N1M0$
  - Stage IVB – $T_{any}N_{any}M1$

Combined Anatomic and Functional Staging

- An important limitation of the AJCC/UICC TNM system is that it does not account for the degree of coexisting liver dysfunction that is present in many patients with HCC. It is well known that a poorer baseline level of hepatic reserve negatively impacts outcomes, even in patients with a low tumor burden.[2] As a result, multiple staging systems have been developed that incorporate anatomic and functional variables.

*Okuda System (**Table 4.3**)*

- The proportion of liver replaced by tumor, ascites, and serum bilirubin and albumin levels were identified as key variables associated with prognosis.[13]
- This system is most applicable to untreated patients, for whom survival times of 8.3, 2.0, and 0.7 months were documented for stage I, II, and III disease, respectively.

Table 4.3   The Okuda Staging System

Points	Tumor/Liver Volume	Clinical Ascites	Albumin	Bilirubin
0	< 50%	Absent	> 3.0 g/dL	≤ 3 mg/dL
1	≥ 50%	Present	≤ 3.0 g/dL	> 3 mg/dL

Stage 1 = 0 points; Stage 2 = 1–2 points; Stage 3 = 3–4 points.

Barcelona Clinical Liver Cancer (BCLC)
*Staging Classification (**Figure 4.1**)*[14]

▦ This is an algorithmic schema that separates patients
into four stages (A, B, C, and D) based on Child-Pugh
score and performance status. The groups are further
subdivided using pathologic features such as the number and size of lesions and the presence of portal venous
invasion. Stage-specific treatments based on the current
standard of care are suggested, along with an estimate of
life expectancy.[14]

▦ The BCLC system has been validated in two prospective studies of patients undergoing treatment for various
stages of HCC.

   ◦ In an American cohort of 239 consecutive HCC
   patients seen over a three year period, the BCLC
   outperformed the TNM, Okuda, Japan Integrated
   Staging (JIS), Chinese University Prognostic Index
   (CUPI), Cancer of the Liver Italian Program (CLIP),
   and Groupe d'Etude et de Traitement du Carcinome
   Hepatocellulaire (GETCH) systems (see below).[15]

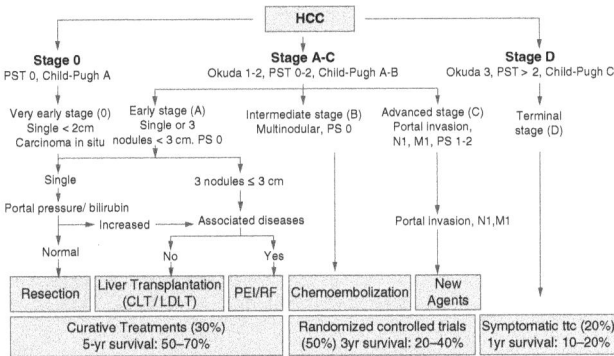

Figure 4.1   The BCLC Algorithm

CLT, cadaveric liver transplantation; LDLT, living donor liver transplantation; PEI, percutaneous ethanol injection; PST/PS, performance status; RF,
radiofrequency ablation; ttc, treatment.

Source: Pons F, Varela M, Llovet JM. Staging systems in hepatocellular carcinoma. *HPB* 2005;7:35–41.

Compared to the other systems, the BCLC had better discriminatory properties, showed the highest homogeneity among patients within the same stage, and was the only staging system shown to independently predict survival. These findings were maintained even after favorable prognosis transplanted patients were excluded.[15]

- Similarly, in an Italian validation cohort of 195 patients, most of whom underwent surgery, the BCLC best predicted survival when compared to the Okuda, JIS, CLIP systems. It also showed superior prognostic power compared to the sixth edition TNM system. Median survival for patients with BCLC stages A, B, C, and D disease was 53, 16, 7, and 3 months, respectively.[16]

- Despite these results, the discriminatory capacity of the BCLC system for patients with advanced (i.e., recurrent, metastatic, unresectable) HCC has been challenged.
  - BCLC stage C disease encompasses those with portal invasion and nodal or distant metastases.[14] By definition, this includes patients with stage IIIB/IVA/IVB disease according to the seventh edition of the AJCC/UICC TNM staging system. The stage groupings AJCC seventh edition were recently modified to reflect the differential prognoses of these anatomic definitions.[11]
  - In a recent retrospective review, the prognostic power of the BCLC system for patients with advanced (BCLC stage C) disease was inferior compared to the CUPI, CLIP, and GETCH systems.[17] The BCLC system is currently being revised in order to address the heterogeneity within this patient population.[18]

Cancer of the Liver Italian Program (CLIP) Score (*Table 4.4*)

- The CLIP score integrates tumor morphology, portal vein thrombosis, and serum α-fetoprotein (AFP) level, in addition to Child-Pugh class. Each covariate is assigned 0 to 2 points depending on the severity, and the sum is then used to assign a prognostic index ranging from 0 to 6.[19]

Table 4.4   The Cancer of the Liver Italian Program (CLIP) Scoring System

Points	Tumor Morphology	Child-Pugh Class	AFP	Portal Vein Thrombosis
0	Uninodular, involves ≤ 50% of liver	A	< 400 ng/dL	No
1	Multinodular, involves ≤ 50% of liver	B	≥ 400 ng/dL	Yes
2	Massive, involves > 50% of liver	C		

▪ The CLIP score was prospectively compared to the Okuda system in a cohort of patients enrolled onto a study of palliative tamoxifen versus best supportive care.[20,21] Eighty-six percent of patients were infected with hepatitis C, 46% had Child-Pugh A cirrhosis, 21% had portal vein thrombosis, and 44% underwent prior locoregional therapy.[21] The CLIP score had better discriminatory power, identifying a subpopulation with a better prognosis within the Okuda stage I group. It also had better predictive power for survival regardless of whether or not patients had previously received locoregional therapy.[21]

▪ The CLIP score was also validated in populations in which the predominant causes of cirrhosis were alcohol and hepatitis B, demonstrating improved prognostic power over the Okuda and BCLC systems.[22,23] Its predictive power appears to be enhanced when performance status is considered.[22]

▪ The CLIP score demonstrated good prognostic power among patients with advanced HCC.[17] Additional variables such as performance status, abdominal pain, aspartate aminotransferase level, and esophageal varices enhanced the CLIP's prognostic power in this population.

▪ Recently, circulating levels of vascular endothelial growth factor (VEGF) were shown to improve the prognostic precision of the CLIP score (i.e., V-CLIP). This tool requires prospective validation.[24]

Japan Integrated Staging (JIS) System

- The JIS system was developed to further refine the discriminative capacity of the CLIP system in patients with low scores (i.e., earlier stage disease).[25]
- The two variables used in the JIS are the Child-Pugh score and TNM stage using the Liver Cancer Study Group of Japan (LCSGJ) criteria. Points are assigned to each variable as follows:
  - Child-Pugh A (0 points), Child-Pugh B (1 point), Child-Pugh C (2 points)
  - LCSGJ Stage I (0 point), Stage II (1 point), Stage III (2 points), Stage IV (3 points)
  - The sum of the points determines the JIS score:
    - JIS 0 – 0 points
    - JIS 1 – 1 point
    - JIS 2 – 2 points
    - JIS 3 – 3 points, etc to a maximum score of 5
- The LCSGJ TNM staging system is based on whether the disease meets the following criteria: (1) solitary tumor; (2) no vascular invasion and (3) a maximum tumor diameter < 2 cm. The presence or absence of lymph node (N0 vs. N1) or distant metastases (M0 vs. M1) are also used for stage classification.
  - T stage:
    - T1 – all 3 criteria met
    - T2 – 2 criteria met
    - T3 – 1 criterion met
    - T4 – 0 criteria met
  - Stage groupings:
    - Stage I – T1N0M0
    - Stage II – T1N0M0
    - Stage III – T3N0N0
    - Stage IVA – T4N0M0, $T_{any}N+M0$
    - Stage IVB – $T_{any}N_{any}M1$
- Although the JIS was shown to have better predictive efficacy over the CLIP, its applicability and practicality may be limited by the use of the rather complex LCSGJ

TNM system. Furthermore, the JIS requires external validation and has not been tested in Western populations.

Chinese University Prognostic Index (CUPI; *Table 4.5*)

▦ The CUPI is composed of six weighted covariates: the presence of symptomatic versus asymptomatic disease; TNM stage; and markers of liver dysfunction including total bilirubin, AFP, alkaline phosphatase (ALP), and ascites. A strength of the CUPI is its weighted scoring system for the different variables. The sum of the scores classifies patients into one of three different risk categories.[26]

▦ The CUPI development and validation cohorts were derived from a purely Chinese patient population seen at a single institution between 1996 and 1998.[27]

  ● Median survival times were 10.1, 3.7, and 1.4 months for the low-, intermediate-, and high-risk groups, respectively.

  ● The CUPI was superior at predicting survival outcomes in this selected population compared to the TNM, Okuda, and CLIP systems.[26]

Table 4.5   The Chinese University Prognostic Index (CUPI)

CUPI Variable	Weighted Score
TNM Stage	
I/II	−3
IIIA/IIIB	−1
IVA/IVB (reference)	0
Asymptomatic disease	−4
Ascites	3
AFP ≥ 500 ng/mL	2
Total Bilirubin (µmol/L or mg/dL)	
< 34 equivalent to <1.9 mg/dL	0
34–51 equivalent to 1.9–2.8 mg/dL	3
≥ 52 equivalent to ≥ 2.9 mg/dL	4
ALP ≥ 200 IU/L	3

Low risk = −7 to 1; intermediate risk = 2–7; high risk = 8–12.

- Compared to the TNM system, the CUPI better predicted survival within the first few months following a diagnosis of HCC. This feature enables the identification of patients most likely to live long enough to benefit from active therapy as opposed to best supportive care.[26]
- The poor performance of the CLIP score in the CUPI population highlighted the limitations of applying some staging systems to populations different from the ones in which they were developed.[27] Eighty-six percent of patients in the CLIP validation cohort had hepatitis C cirrhosis, whereas 80% of the CUPI population had hepatitis B cirrhosis.[21,26]
- In the retrospective review evaluating the optimal staging system for a North American patient cohort with advanced HCC, the CUPI demonstrated good prognostic efficacy. This patient population included equal proportions of patients with hepatitis B, hepatitis C, and alcoholic cirrhosis (approximately 30% each).[17]
- The CUPI awaits prospective external validation, and its generalizability to other ethnic groups and etiologies of cirrhosis will need to be further investigated.

Groupe d'Etude et de Traitement du Carcinome Hepatocellulaire (GETCH; *Table 4.6*)

- The GETCH system was developed and validated in a cohort of 761 patients representing 24 Western medical centers.[28]
- Key prognostic variables identified were Karnofsky performance status (KPS), serum bilirubin, alkaline phosphatase (ALP), AFP, and ultrasonographic evidence of portal venous obstruction.[29]
- The covariates are scored using a points system, and the sum of the points divides patients into three risk groups: A (0 points, low risk of death), B (1–5 points, intermediate risk), and C (≥ 6 points, high risk).
  - These risk groups corresponded to significant differences in 1-year survival: 72%, 34%, and 7% for group A, B, and C, respectively.[29]
  - The GETCH system also requires external validation.

Table 4.6   Groupe d'Etude et de Traitement du Carcinome Hepatocellulaire (GETCH) System

Points	KPS	Serum Bilirubin	ALP	AFP	Portal Vein Thrombosis
0	≥ 80%	< 50 µmol/L *or* < 2.9 mg/dL	< 2 × ULN	< 35 µg/L	No
1					Yes
2			≥ 2 × ULN	≥ 35 µg/L	
3	< 80%	≥ 50 µmol/L *or* > 2.9 µg/dL			

ULN, upper limit of normal.

Issues and Controversies

▪ The multitude of available staging systems, each with their own strengths and limitations, creates a quandary for the clinician in deciding which system is the most comprehensive and accurate for day-to-day clinical practice. In addition, the fact that many of these systems were developed in patient populations that differed by ethnicity, underlying etiology of liver disease, and disease extent limits their applicability and comparability.

▪ For routine clinical practice, the AJCC/UICC TNM system is still used given its familiarity and easy translatability across the different specialists in a multidisciplinary cancer care team as well as globally. The sixth edition is the only system to have been validated for patients undergoing liver transplantation for the primary treatment of HCC.[11] The updated seventh edition provides an HCC-specific staging classification and recognizes the differential impact of portal vein thrombosis and lymph node metastases on prognosis.

▪ The question of which staging systems are most applicable for patients with advanced, unresectable HCC was recently addressed in a review conducted at Memorial

Sloan-Kettering Cancer Center. Of the seven different staging systems, the GETCH, CLIP, and CUPI systems were found to have the best prognostic accuracy for this patient population.[17]

- Although the BCLC system is a practical algorithm that provides both staging and management information, this system is inadequate for prognostication in patients with advanced HCC.[17] This is mainly due to the heterogeneous composition of patients with stage C disease, which limits its discriminatory capacity among patients whose disease is not resectable, but who are still well enough for systemic therapy. This issue is currently being reevaluated.[18]

- A unified, internationally validated classification scheme may help to optimize the care of patients with HCC. However, it is unclear whether this will be feasible considering the different outcomes governed by the different etiologies of the disease. Furthermore, as new targeted therapies emerge based on new discoveries into the molecular pathogenesis of HCC, it can be expected that genetic signatures will eventually be incorporated into staging systems, potentially increasing their precision but also their complexity.

■ Prognostic Factors

- In addition to stage, other factors have prognostic importance in HCC.

Variant Estrogen Receptor (ER) Status

- A variant ER transcript containing an exon 5 deletion was identified in men who developed HCC.[29] Variant ERs remain constitutively active and have an altered hormone binding domain, which may explain why trials of tamoxifen have not shown consistent benefit in HCC.[29–31] Variant ER status is associated with more aggressive disease biology and has been shown to be a stronger predictor of poor prognosis than the CLIP and BCLC stage.[32]

Histopathology

- Encapsulated tumors and the fibrolamellar variant of HCC (see Chapter 5: Histopathology) are associated with more favorable outcomes.[33,34]
- The degree of fibrosis has been shown to adversely affect survival outcomes irrespective of the AJCC/UICC TNM stage.[35] Documentation of the fibrosis (F) score (F0 = 0–4 or none to moderate fibrosis; F1 = 5–6 or severe fibrosis to cirrhosis) is recommended by the AJCC, but it is not a formal part of the staging system.[12,35]

Serum AFP Levels

- Although false-negative results can occur, especially in small early-stage tumors, AFP levels have been shown to correlate strongly with disease burden for tumors > 3 cm in diameter.[36,37]
- Elevated AFP levels also correlate with poorly differentiated histology and decreased survival.[38,39]

Hepatitis B Virus (HBV) and Hepatitis C Virus (HCV) Infection

- In both Asian and Western series, HCC patients infected with HCV experience a significantly shorter disease-free survival following surgery than their HBV-infected counterparts.[40,41] This is likely related to the presence of cirrhosis as well as a more aggressive disease biology characterized by poor differentiation and a higher incidence of vascular invasion.[41]
- Data are conflicting as to the effect of HBV on prognosis after hepatectomy.[42,43] Patients with serologic evidence of ongoing viral replication (i.e., envelope antigen positive) appear to have a worse prognosis.[44,45]

Molecular Markers

- MicroRNAs are short, noncoding RNA molecules that regulate gene expression, are tumor specific, and have been implicated in hepatocarcinogenesis.[46,47] MicroRNAs have also been shown to have predictive and prognostic potential.

- *miR-26* was found to be differentially expressed between men and women and distinguished between tumor versus normal tissue. Decreased *miR-26* expression was associated with malignant tumors and a shorter survival time but was also associated with better responses to interferon therapy.[47]
- Elevated circulating levels of VEGF (> 450 pg/mL) were recently shown to be an independent predictor of poor survival. As previously mentioned, the addition of serum VEGF to the CLIP scoring system (V-CLIP) improved its prognostic power.[24]
- *c-MET* is a receptor tyrosine kinase that binds *hepatocyte growth factor (HGF)* to control normal organogenesis and morphogenesis.[48]
  - Overexpression of *c-MET* has been found in up to 50% of HCC tumors.[49] This has been associated with earlier stage tumors with favorable prognostic features.[50]
  - The impact of *c-MET* overexpression on prognosis is unclear as data are conflicting.[50–52]
- Other types of molecular and gene expression studies including the use of markers of inflammation, fractional allelic imbalance, and genomics analysis show great potential for providing prognostic information for patients who have undergone liver transplantation for HCC.[53]

Geography and Ethnicity

- Patients with HCC from high-incidence areas such as sub-Saharan Africa and Asia have been observed to have a shorter survival time than patients from low-incidence, Western countries. They are also more likely to present with metastases than their Western counterparts. Differences in risk factors, environment, genetics, and access to health care are likely at play.[54]

■ References

1. Abou-Alfa GK. Hepatocellular carcinoma: molecular biology and therapy. *Semin Oncol* 2006;33(6 Suppl 11):S79–S83.
2. Poon RT, Fan ST, Lo CM, et al. Long-term prognosis after resection of hepatocellular carcinoma associated with hepatitis B-related cirrhosis. *J Clin Oncol* 2000;18:1094–1101.

3. Child CG III, Turcotte JG. Surgery and portal hypertension. In: Child CG III (ed). *The Liver and Portal Hypertension* Philadelphia: WB Saunders, 1964:50.
4. Pugh RN, Murray-Lyon IM, Dawson JL, et al. Transection of the oesophagus for bleeding oesophageal varices. *Br J Surg* 1973;60:646–649.
5. de Franchis R, Primignani M. Why do varices bleed? *Gastroenterol Clin North Am* 1992;21:85–101.
6. Garrison RN, Cryer HM, Howard DA, et al. Clarification of risk factors for abdominal operations in patients with hepatic cirrhosis. *Ann Surg* 1984;199:648–655.
7. Albers I, Hartmann H, Bircher J, et al. Superiority of the Child-Pugh classification to quantitative liver function tests for assessing prognosis of liver cirrhosis. *Scand J Gastroenterol* 1989;24:269–276.
8. Durand F, Valla D. Assessment of the prognosis of cirrhosis: Child-Pugh versus MELD. *J Hepatol* 2005;42:S100–S107.
9. Kamath PS, Wiesner RH, Malinchoc M, et al. A model to predict survival in patients with end-stage liver disease. *Hepatology* 2001;33:464–470.
10. Wiesner R, Edwards E, Freeman R, et al. Model for end-stage liver disease (MELD) and allocation of donor livers. *Gastroenterology* 2003;124:91–96.
11. Vauthey JN, Ribero D, Abdalla EK, et al. Outcomes of liver transplantation in 490 patients with hepatocellular carcinoma: validation of a uniform staging after surgical treatment. *J Am Coll Surg* 2007;204:1016–1027.
12. Liver. In: Edge SB, Byrd DR, Compton CC, et al (eds). *AJCC Cancer Staging Handbook*. 7th ed. New York: Springer, 2010: 237–245.
13. Okuda K, Ohtsuki T, Obata H, et al. Natural history of hepatocellular carcinoma and prognosis in relation to treatment. Study of 850 patients. *Cancer* 1985;56:918–928.
14. Llovet JM, Bru C, Bruix J. Prognosis of hepatocellular carcinoma: the BCLC staging classification. *Semin Liver Dis* 1999; 19:329–338.
15. Marrero JA, Fontana RJ, Barrat A, et al. Prognosis of hepatocellular carcinoma: comparison of 7 staging systems in an American cohort. *Hepatology* 2005;41:707–716.
16. Cillo U, Vitale A, Grigoletto F, et al. Prospective validation of the Barcelona Clinic Liver Cancer staging system. *J Hepatol* 2006;44:723–731.
17. Huitzil-Melendez F-D, Capanu M, O'Reilly EM, et al. Advanced hepatocellular carcinoma: which staging system best predicts prognosis? *J Clin Oncol* 2010;28:2889–2895.
18. Llovet JM. Presented at the State of Clinical Science Meeting. Statement at the State of the Clinical Science

Meeting: Hepatocellular Carcinoma (HCC). December 12–13, 2008, Bethesda, MD.

19. Cancer of the Liver Italian Program (CLIP) Investigators. A new prognostic system for hepatocellular carcinoma: a retrospective study of 435 patients. *Hepatology* 1998;28:751–755.

20. CLIP Group (Cancer of the Liver Italian Program). Tamoxifen in the treatment of hepatocellular carcinoma: a randomised controlled trial. *Lancet* 1998;352:17–20.

21. The Cancer of the Liver Italian Program (CLIP) Investigators. Prospective validation of the CLIP score: a new prognostic system for patients with cirrhosis and hepatocellular carcinoma. *Hepatology* 2000;31:840–845.

22. Collette S, Bonnetain F, Paoletti X, et al. Prognosis of advanced hepatocellular carcinoma: comparison of three staging systems in two French clinical trials. *Ann Oncol* 2008; 19:1117–1126.

23. Levy I, Sherman M. Staging of hepatocellular carcinoma: assessment of the CLIP, Okuda, and Child-Pugh staging systems in a cohort of 257 patients in Toronto. *Gut* 2002; 50:881–885.

24. Kaseb AO, Hassan M, Lin E, et al. Effect of incorporating plasma VEGF level into a v-CLIP scoring system on stratification of patients with hepatocellular carcinoma. 2010 Gastrointestinal Cancers Symposium, Orlando, FL, Abstract 155.

25. Kudo M, Chung H, Osaki Y. Prognostic staging system for hepatocellular carcinoma (CLIP score): its value and limitations, and a proposal of a new staging system, the Japan Integrated Staging Score (JIS score). *J Gastroenterol* 2003;38:207–215.

26. Leung T, Tang A, Zee B, et al. Construction of the Chinese University Prognostic Index for hepatocellular carcinoma and comparison with the TNM staging system, the Okuda staging system, and the Cancer of the Liver Italian Program staging system. A study based on 926 patients. *Cancer* 2002; 94:1760–1769.

27. Abou-Alfa GK, Huitzil-Melendez FD, O'Reilly EM, et al. Current management of advanced hepatocellular carcinoma. *Gastrointest Cancer Res* 2008;2:64–70.

28. Chevret S, Trinchet JC, Mathieu D, et al. A new prognostic classification for predicting survival in patients with hepatocellular carcinoma. Groupe d'Etude et de Traitement du Carcinome Hepatocellulaire. *J Hepatol* 1999;31:133–141.

29. Villa E, Camellini L, Dugani A, et al. Variant estrogen receptor messenger RNA species detected in human primary hepatocellular carcinoma. *Cancer Res* 1995;55:498–500.

30. Martinez-Cereso FJ, Tomas A, Enriquez J, et al. Tamoxifen improves survival in patients with advanced hepatocellular carcinoma. *J Hepatol* 1991;13(Suppl):S51.

31. Villa E, Dugani A, Fantoni E, et al. Type of estrogen receptor determines response to antiestrogen therapy in hepatocellular carcinoma. *Cancer Res* 1996;56:3883–3885.

32. Villa E, Colantoni A, Camma C, et al. Estrogen receptor classification for hepatocellular carcinoma: comparison with clinical staging systems. *J Clin Oncol* 2003;21:441–446.

33. Stipa F, Yoon SS, Liau KH, et al. Outcome of patients with fibrolamellar hepatocellular carcinoma. *Cancer* 2006;106: 1331–1338.

34. Okuda K, Musha H, Nakajima Y, et al. Clinicopathologic features of encapsulated hepatocellular carcinoma: a study of 26 cases. *Cancer* 1977;40:1240–1245.

35. Ishak K, Baptista A, Bianchi L, et al. Histological grading and staging of chronic hepatitis. *J Hepatol* 1995;22:696–699.

36. Chen DS, Sung JL, Sheu JC, et al. Serum alpha-fetoprotein in the early stage of human hepatocellular carcinoma. *Gastroenterology* 1984;86:1404–1409.

37. Ebara M, Ohto M, Shinagawa T, et al. Natural history of minute hepatocellular carcinoma smaller than three centimeters complicating cirrhosis. A study in 22 patients. *Gastroenterology* 1986;90:289–298.

38. Tangkijvanich P, Anukulkarnkusol N, Suwangool P, et al. Clinical characteristics and prognosis of hepatocellular carcinoma: analysis based on serum alpha-fetoprotein levels. *J Clin Gastroenterol* 2000;31:302–308.

39. Matsumoto Y, Suzuki T, Asada I, et al. Clinical classification of hepatoma in Japan according to serial changes in serum alpha-fetoprotein levels. *Cancer* 1982;49:354–360.

40. Sasaki Y, Yamada T, Tanaka H, et al. Risk of recurrence in a long-term follow-up after surgery in 417 patients with hepatitis B- or hepatitis C-related hepatocellular carcinoma. *Ann Surg* 2006;244:771–780.

41. Roayaie S, Haim MB, Emre S, et al. Comparison of surgical outcomes for hepatocellular carcinoma in patients with hepatitis B versus hepatitis C: a Western experience. *Ann Surg Oncol* 2000;7:764–770.

42. Poon RT, Fan ST, Lo CM, et al. Long-term prognosis after resection of hepatocellular carcinoma associated with hepatitis B-related cirrhosis. *J Clin Oncol* 2000;18:1094–1101.

43. Cescon M, Cucchetti A, Grazi GL, et al. Role of hepatitis B virus infection in the prognosis after hepatectomy for hepatocellular carcinoma in patients with cirrhosis: a Western dual-center experience. *Arch Surg* 2009;144:906–913.

44. Sun HC, Zhang W, Qin LX, et al. Positive serum hepatitis B e antigen is associated with higher risk of early recurrence and poorer survival in patients after curative resection of hepatitis B-related hepatocellular carcinoma. *J Hepatol* 2007;47:684–690.

45. Kubo S, Hirohashi K, Yamazaki O, et al. Effect of the presence of hepatitis B e antigen on prognosis after liver resection for hepatocellular carcinoma in patients with chronic hepatitis B. *World J Surg* 2002;26:555–560.
46. Huang S, He X. The role of microRNAs in liver progression. *Br J Cancer* 2011;104:235–240.
47. Junfang J, Jiong S, Budhu A, et al. MicroRNA expression, survival, and response to interferon in liver cancer. *N Engl J Med* 2009;361:1437–1447.
48. Matsomoto K, Nakamura T. Emerging multipotent aspects of hepatocyte growth factor. *J Biochem* 1996;119:591–600.
49. Boix L, Rosa JL, Ventura F, et al. c-MET mRNA overexpression in human hepatocellular carcinoma. *Hepatology* 1994;19:88–91.
50. Huitzil FD, Sun MY, Capanu M, et al. Expression of the c-met and HGF in resected hepatocellular carcinoma (rHCC): correlation with clinicopathological features (CP) and overall survival (OS) [abstract]. *J Clin Oncol* 2008;26(Suppl):4599.
51. Kaposi-Novak P, Lee JS, Gomez-Quiroz L, et al. Met-regulated expression signature defines a subset of human hepatocellular carcinomas with poor prognosis and aggressive phenotype. *J Clin Invest* 2006;116:1582–1595.
52. Ueki T, Fujimoto J, Suzuki T, et al. Expression of hepatocyte growth factor and its receptor, the c-met proto-oncogene, in hepatocellular carcinoma. *Hepatology* 1997;25:619–623.
53. Schmidt C, Marsh JW. Molecular signature for HCC: role in predicting outcomes after liver transplant and selection for potential adjuvant treatment. *Curr Opin Organ Transpl* 2010;15:277–282.
54. Artinyan A, Mailey B, Sanchez-Luege N, et al. Race, ethnicity and socioeconomic status influence the survival of patients with hepatocellular carcinoma in the United States. *Cancer* 2010;116:1367–1377.

Histopathology

■ Introduction

Pathologic examination of liver tumor tissue provides valuable diagnostic and prognostic information that can help to guide therapy and predict outcomes. Although several histologic subtypes of liver tumors exist, this chapter will focus on malignant and benign hepatocellular liver tumors.

■ Malignant Hepatocellular Liver Tumors

Hepatocellular Carcinoma (HCC)

- HCC cells are larger than normal hepatocytes and contain large nucleoli with a high nuclear:cytoplasmic ratio. Nuclear irregularity and hyperchromatism are occasionally observed.[1] (See **Figure 5.1**[1]).
- The cytoplasm is typically eosinophilic (pink) and finely granular from the presence of hyaline globules containing α-1-antitrypsin, fibrinogen, and other plasma proteins. Fat and glycogen content may impart a whitish, clear cell appearance.[1] These fatty changes occur in up to 40% of small (< 2 cm in diameter), well-differentiated tumors, but diminish as they grow and dedifferentiate.[2,3] Eosinophilic, "twisted-rope" inclusions known as Mallory-Denk bodies may also be present and are associated with alcoholic and metabolic causes of chronic liver disease.[4] (See **Figure 5.2**.[1]) The cellular growth pattern often resembles that of normal liver parenchyma, forming trabeculae separated by venous sinusoids with interspersed biliary canaliculi containing bile pigment.

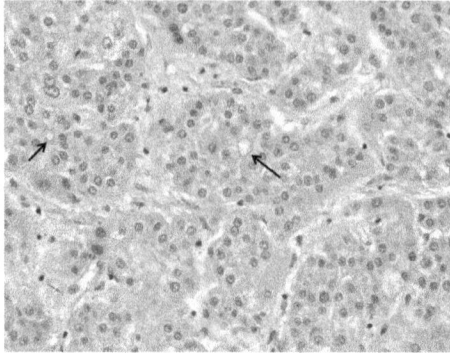

Figure 5.1   Hepatocellular Carcinoma Cells with Eosinophilic Cytoplasm and a High Nuclear:Cytoplasmic Ratio

Source: Courtesy of Rachel Hudacko, MD; Department of Pathology, MSKCC. Arrows indicate bile canaliculi.

Growth pattern variations include a pseudoglandular arrangement with trabeculae separated by dilated canaliculi or a compact arrangement of trabecular sheets and compressed sinusoids.[1]

■ The absence of desmoplastic stromal invasion is a key distinguishing characteristic that is unique to HCC, although a scirrhous subtype exists that has profuse stroma.[1,5]

■ Although no single immunohistochemical stain consistently and reliably distinguishes HCC from other

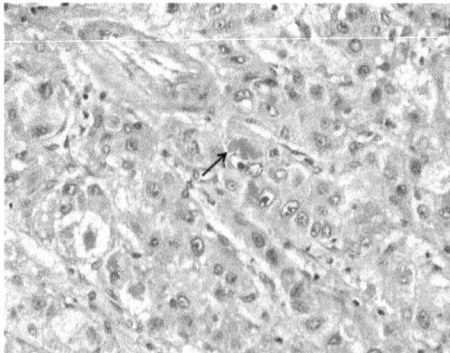

Figure 5.2   Mallory-Denk Cytoplasmic Inclusion Bodies

Source: Courtesy of Rachel Hudacko, MD; Department of Pathology, MSKCC.

malignant or benign liver lesions, certain markers may help to narrow the differential, when interpreted within the appropriate clinical context.

- Hepatocyte paraffin-1 (HepPar-1): This liver mito-chondrial stain is positive in about 90% of HCC cases but is also found in approximately 4% of cholangiocar-cinomas and metastatic adenocarcinomas.[6,7]
- Polyclonal CD34: This endothelial marker is usually negative in normal hepatic sinusoidal endothelium. The staining pattern of CD34 may help to distinguish HCC from benign liver lesions such as cirrhotic nod-ules, but this is highly variable.[1,8]
- Polyclonal carcinoembryonic antigen (pCEA) stains bile canaliculi in both normal liver and HCC, but not liver metastases.[9]
- Tumor α-fetoprotein (AFP) positivity can be helpful, but only occurs in 50% of cases.[1]
- Cytokeratins including CK7, CK20, and AE1/AE3 have limited utility in HCC.[1]

- In addition to these "traditional" immunohistochemical stains, several new markers have been identified:
  - Glypican-3 (GPC3) is a heparan sulfate proteoglycan that is elevated in the serum of patients with HCC, but not in healthy patients or those with benign liver disease. A recent series reported that GPC3 immuno-reactivity had a sensitivity and specificity of 83% and 100%, respectively, for identifying HCC tumors and distinguishing them from other liver lesions including cholangiocarcinomas and metastases.[10]
  - Heat shock protein-70 (HSP70) is an antiapoptotic fac-tor that is upregulated in HCC.[11] In one series, HSP70 immunoreactivity distinguished HCC from nonmalig-nant nodules with a sensitivity and specificity of 74% and 98%, respectively. The positive and negative predic-tive values were 98% and 79%, respectively.[12]
  - Glutamine synthetase (GS) is involved in glutamine pro-duction, an important energy source for tumor cells.[13] MicroRNA overexpression of GS occurs in HCC, and GS immunoreactivity progressively increases as hepato-cytes assume a more malignant phenotype.[14,15]

• GPC3, HSP70, and GS have remarkable discriminative potential when used in combination. All three
markers were shown to be present in approximately
50% of early, low-grade HCCs and 0% of dysplastic
nodules. Conversely, the absence of all three occurred
in 73% of dysplastic nodules but only 3% of early, low-
grade HCCs. Immunoreactivity for two out of three
markers had the best sensitivity and specificity for distinguishing low-grade HCC from dysplastic nodules,
at 72% and 100%, respectively.[12]

Fibrolamellar Hepatocellular Carcinoma (FLL-HCC)

▓ FLL-HCC represents only 0.9% of all primary liver tumors,[16] but represents an important diagnostic distinc-
tion given its clinical and practical implications.

▓ Tumors consist of large polygonal cells with abundant
granular, eosinophilic cytoplasm surrounded by thick
fibrous bands.[17]

▓ Tumors may demonstrate immunoreactivity for HepPar-1
and CD99.[18,19] Carcinoembryonic antigen (CEA), α-1-
antitrypsin, fibrinogen, and copper are also present at
higher levels in FLL-HCC than in traditional HCC.[20]

▓ Biliary markers including cytokeratins 7 and 19, epithe-
lial membrane antigen (EMA), and EpCAM may also
be present.[21] Some tumors stain for neuroendocrine
markers.[22–23]

Mixed Cholangiocarcinoma-Hepatocellular Carcinoma

▓ Poorly differentiated HCC can be very difficult to distinguish from a poorly differentiated intrahepatic
cholangiocarcinoma.

▓ Lesions with abundant stroma and lacking markers of
hepatocellular differentiation (i.e., granular HepPar-1
staining, trabecular growth pattern, positive AFP, bile
canaliculi) suggest an adenocarcinoma.

▓ Well-differentiated cholangiocarcinoma cells display
a columnar or cuboidal morphology and, unlike HCC

cells, have small nucleoli. Architecturally, the cells are arranged in tubules and glands but can also form nests, cords, papillae, or a cribriform growth pattern. Abundant mucin may be present.

- Cytoplasmic immunoreactivity for CEA and pancytokeratins AE1/AE3 is common.[1]

Hepatoblastoma

- Hepatoblastomas represent 80% of all primary pediatric liver tumors.[24]
- Risk factors include low birth weight, Beckwith-Wiedemann syndrome, familial adenomatous polyposis, and chronic cholestasis syndromes.[25–27]
- These heterogeneous tumors contain semi-differentiated fetal and embryonal hepatoblasts, which are smaller and have a higher nuclear:cytoplasmic ratio than normal hepatocytes. Fetal hepatoblasts may contain cytoplasmic fat and/or glycogen deposits. Both cell types are capable of extramedullary hematopoiesis. Mesenchymal and neuroectodermal elements may be present.[28]
- Surgical resection, where possible, produces the best outcomes. Advanced disease is treated with cisplatin ± doxorubicin–based chemotherapy.[28]

Carcinosarcoma

- Hepatic carcinosarcomas are extremely rare liver tumors; only 20 cases have been reported in the English literature.[29]
- These are hybrids of hepatocellular or cholangiocarcinoma cells and sarcomatous cells.[30]
- These are believed to arise from the metaplastic transformation of carcinomatous cells into sarcomatous cells.[31]
- The clinical profile of patients with carcinosarcoma appears to be similar to that of HCC: older, male, with underlying liver cirrhosis.[29]
- Hepatic carcinosarcomas behave aggressively and present with widespread metastases at diagnosis. In one series, most patients died within 6 months of palliative surgery, although long-term survivors have also been reported.[29]

■ Benign Hepatocellular Liver Tumors

Dysplastic Nodules

- These are benign but premalignant lesions that eventually evolve into HCC.

Low-Grade Dysplastic Nodules (L-DN)

- These are often characterized by large dysplastic or atypical cells that usually contain normal cytoplasm, although diffuse siderosis and increased copper content are occasionally present.[32]
- Cells grow more densely than neighboring cirrhotic hepatocytes and are contained within a fibrous pseudocapsule but are not distinctly nodular. Regenerative changes may be seen. Small "unpaired" arteries unaccompanied by bile ducts represent neovascularization.[33]
- Currently, L-DNs cannot be distinguished from regenerative nodules, but this difference is not known to be clinically significant.[3]

High-Grade Dysplastic Nodules (H-DN)

- Unlike L-DNs, H-DNs exhibit small-cell dysplasia or atypia with features suggestive of increased cell proliferation such as a high nuclear:cytoplasmic ratio.[1,34]
- Architecturally, H-DNs have a denser and more nodular appearance than L-DNs, may grow in trabecular cords, and display a higher frequency of unpaired arteries. Small, separate, dysplastic foci may also be observed. Occasionally, H-DNs contain subnodules with a high proliferative index that represent early, well-differentiated HCC in what is known as a "nodule-in-nodule."[3,35]
- H-DNs are differentiated from HCC by the presence of stromal invasion that is immunoreactive for cytokeratins 7 and 19.[36] Stromal invasion is absent in true HCC.
- The classification of borderline or equivocal nodules differs between Asian and Western pathologists; nodules typically classified by Asian pathologists as early, well-differentiated HCC are often declared as H-DNs by Western pathologists.[37] The correct diagnosis hinges on a thorough review of the pathologic findings as well as the clinical course.

- Approximately one third of H-DNs evolve into HCC.[38,39] Surgical and nonsurgical ablative procedures such as percutaneous ethanol injection or thermal ablation may be considered as preventive measures, but each has its own limitations, and there is currently no standard approach.[40,41]

Hepatocellular Adenoma (HCA)

- A benign lesion arising from normal liver parenchyma in a woman of reproductive age and a history of prolonged oral contraceptive pill (OCP) use is pathognomonic of HCA.[42] The relationship between OCP use and HCA is so robust that alternative diagnoses such as focal nodular hyperplasia or well-differentiated HCC must be considered in patients who do not fit this profile.[1]
- Men who take anabolic steroids may also develop HCAs.[43,44]
- Presenting symptoms include chronic abdominal pain due to mass effect because HCAs usually average 5–15 cm in diameter, but can span up to 30 cm. Acute abdominal pain may occur due to rupture and hemorrhage of large HCAs.[44,45]
- HCA cells contain benign hepatocytes with a normal nuclear:cytoplasmic ratio and no mitoses. Cells are often arranged in sheets and cords, and bile ducts are absent. Surrounding cells are typically larger and paler due to increased fat and/or glycogen content.[1]
- On unenhanced computed tomography (CT) scans, HCAs are discrete, iso- or hyperdense lesions.[46] On triphasic CT scans, HCAs exhibit arterial phase iso- or hypoenhancement followed by portal venous phase hyperenhancement.[46,47] The enhancement pattern is inhomogeneous, central scarring is absent, and subcapsular feeding arteries may be seen.[47]
- On gadolinium-enhanced magnetic resonance imaging (MRI), HCA demonstrates hyperenhancement during the arterial phase that quickly falls off during the venous phase. Lesions are hypo- to hyperintense on T1-weighted images and are iso- to hyperintense on T2-weighted images.[48]

- Superparamagnetic iron oxide (SPIO) is a liver-specific contrast agent that is selectively taken up by phagocytic Kupffer cells, which are often absent from malignant tumors. SPIO uptake causes a decreased signal on T2-weighted images, so that malignant tumors appear hyperintense while normal liver and benign lesions such as HCAs appear dark.[49]
- Ultrasonography is a poor diagnostic tool for HCA; sensitivity is only 30%.[50]
- HCAs have malignant potential; 5–10% transform into HCC.[50] The risk is higher in males, tumors > 5 cm, and telangiectatic and unclassified subtypes of HCAs. Surgical resection is a safe and effective preventative measure.[45,51]

Focal Nodular Hyperplasia (FNH)

- FNH is the second most common benign liver tumor after hemangioma and occurs most frequently in women of reproductive age, although it can also be found in men.[52]
- FNH may grow or regress over time but has no known malignant potential.[53,54]
- FNH consists of hepatocytes and Kupffer cells and is believed to represent a reactive lesion that develops in response to vascular injury.[55]
- In contrast to HCA, FNH on triphasic CT scan exhibits a homogenous enhancement pattern, central scarring, but no capsular enhancement due to the absence of subcapsular feeding arteries. FNH also shows greater enhancement during the arterial phase than HCAs.[47] These features are key in helping to distinguish FNH from HCA, HCC, and FLL-HCC.[48]
- FNH is iso- to hypointense on T1-weighted MRI images and is iso- to hyperintense on T2-weighted images.[48]
- Expectant management in asymptomatic patients is appropriate, although minimally invasive liver resection is another option.[56,57]

■ Other Primary Malignant Liver Neoplasms[1]

- Biliary: cholangiocarcinoma, cystadenocarcinoma
- Vascular: angiosarcoma, epithelioid hemangioendothelioma
- Miscellaneous: lymphoma, other rare tumors or sarcomas

■ References

1. Goodman ZD. Neoplasms of the liver. *Mod Pathol* 2007;(20 Suppl 1):S49–S60.

2. Kutami R, Nakashima Y, Nakashima O, et al. Pathomorphologic study on the mechanism of fatty change in small hepatocellular carcinoma of humans. *J Hepatol* 2000;33:282–289.

3. International Consensus Group for Hepatocellular Neoplasia. Pathologic diagnosis of early hepatocellular carcinoma: a report of the international consensus group for hepatocellular neoplasia. *Hepatology* 2009;49:658–664.

4. Strnad P, Zatloukal K, Stumptner C, et al. Mallory-Denk bodies: lessons from keratin-containing hepatic inclusion bodies. *Biochim Biophys Acta* 2008;1782:764–774.

5. Ishak KG, Goodman Z, Stocker J. *Tumors of the Liver and Intrahepatic Bile Ducts. Atlas of Tumor Pathology, Third Series, Fascicle 31.* Washington, DC: Armed Forces Institute of Pathology, 2001.

6. Lugli A, Tornillo L, Mirlacher M, et al. Hepatocyte paraffin 1 expression in human normal and neoplastic tissues: tissue microarray analysis on 3,940 tissue samples. *Am J Clin Pathol* 2004;122:721–727.

7. Minervini MI, Demetris AJ, Lee RG, et al. Utilization of hepatocyte-specific antibody in the immunocytochemical evaluation of liver tumors. *Mod Pathol* 1997;10:686–692.

8. Gouysse G, Frachon S, Hervieu V, et al. Endothelial cell differentiation in hepatocellular adenomas: implications for histopathological diagnosis. *J Hepatol* 2004;41:259–266.

9. Wolber RA, Greene CA, Dupuis BA. Polyclonal carcinoembryonic antigen staining in the cytologic differential diagnosis of primary and metastatic hepatic malignancies. *Acta Cytol* 1991;35:215–220.

10. Wang FH, Yip YC, Zhang M, et al. Diagnostic utility of glypican-3 for hepatocellular carcinoma on liver needle biopsy. *J Clin Pathol* 2010;63:599–603.

11. Chuma M, Sakamoto M, Yamakazi K, et al. Expression profiling in multistage hepatocarcinogenesis: identification of HSP70 as a molecular marker of early hepatocellular carcinoma. *Hepatology* 2003;37:198–207.

12. Di Tommaso L, Franchi G, Park YN, et al. Diagnostic value of HSP70, glypican 3, and glutamine synthetase in hepatocellular nodules in cirrhosis. *Hepatology* 2007;45:725–734.

13. Reitzer LJ, Wice BM, Kennell D. Evidence that glutamine, not sugar, is the major energy source for cultured HeLa cells. *J Biol Chem* 1979;254:2669–2676.

14. Christa L, Simon MT, Flinois JP, et al. Overexpression of glutamine synthetase in human primary liver cancer. *Gastroenterology* 1994;106:1312–1320.

15. Osada T, Sakamoto M, Nagawa H, et al. Acquisition of glutamine synthetase expression in human hepatocarcinogenesis: relation to disease recurrence and possible regulation by ubiquitin-dependent proteolysis. *Cancer* 1999;85:819–831.

16. El-Serag HB, Davila JA. Is fibrolamellar carcinoma different from hepatocellular carcinoma? A US population-based study. *Hepatology* 2004;39:798–803.

17. Craig JR, Peters RL, Edmondson HA, et al. Fibrolamellar carcinoma of the liver: a tumor of adolescents and young adults with distinctive clinicopathologic features. *Cancer* 1980;46:372–379.

18. Klein WM, Molmenti EP, Colombani PM, et al. Primary liver carcinoma arising in people younger than 30 years. *Am J Clin Pathol* 2005;124:512–518.

19. Vasdev N, Nayak NC. CD99 expression in hepatocellular carcinoma: an immunohistochemical study in the fibrolamellar and common variant of the tumour. *Indian J Pathol Microbiol* 2003;46:625–629.

20. Teitelbaum DH, Tuttle S, Carey LC, et al. Fibrolamellar carcinoma of the liver. Review of three cases and the presentation of a characteristic set of tumor markers defining this tumor. *Ann Surg* 1985;202:36–41.

21. Ward SC, Huang J, Tickoo SK, et al. Fibrolamellar hepatocellular carcinoma of the liver exhibits immunohistochemical evidence of both hepatocyte and bile duct differentiation. *Mod Pathol* 2010;23(9):1180–1190

22. Payne CM, Nagle RB, Paplanus SH, Graham AR. Fibrolamellar carcinoma of the liver: a primary malignant oncocytic carcinoid? *Ultrastruct Pathol* 1986;10(6):539–552.

23. Lloreta J, Vadell C, Fabregat X, Serrano S. Fibrolamellar hepatic tumor with neurosecretory features and systemic deposition of AA amyloid. *Ultrastruct Pathol* 1994;18(1-2):287–292.

24. Darbari A, Sabin KM, Shapiro CN, et al. Epidemiology of primary hepatic malignancies in U.S. children. *Hepatology* 2003;38:560–566.

25. Reynolds M, Urayama KY, Von Behren J, et al. Birth characteristics and hepatoblastoma risk in young children. *Cancer* 2004;100:1070–1076.

26. Tan TY, Amor DJ. Tumour surveillance in Beckwith-Wiedemann syndrome and hemihyperplasia: a critical review of the evidence and suggested guidelines for local practice. *J Paediatr Child Health* 2006;42:486–490.

27. Hirschman BA, Pollock BH, Tomlinson GE. The spectrum of APC mutations in children with hepatoblastoma from familial adenomatous polyposis kindreds. *J Pediatr* 2005;147:263–266.

28. Finegold MJ, Egler RA, Goss JA, et al. Liver tumors: pediatric population. *Liver Transpl* 2008;14:1545–1556.

29. Lao XM, Chen DY, Zhang YQ, et al. Primary carcinosarcoma of the liver: clinicopathologic features of 5 cases and a review of the literature. *Am J Surg Pathol* 2007;31:817–826.
30. Ishak KG, Anthony PP, Niederau C, et al. Mesenchymal tumours of the liver. In: Stanley RH, Lauri AA (eds). *WHO International Histological Classification of Tumours, Pathology & Genetics of the Tumours of the Digestive System.* Lyon, France: IARC Press, 2000:198.
31. Kubosawa H, Ishige H, Kondo Y, et al. Hepatocellular carcinoma with rhabdomyoblastic differentiation. *Cancer* 1988;62: 781–786.
32. Anthony PP, Vogel CL, Barker LF. Liver cell dysplasia: a premalignant condition. *J Clin Pathol* 1973;26:217–223.
33. Park YN, Yang CP, Fernandez GJ, et al. Neoangiogenesis and sinusoidal "capillarization" in dysplastic nodules of the liver. *Am J Surg Pathol* 1998;22:656–662.
34. Watanabe S, Okita K, Harada T, et al. Morphologic studies of the liver cell dysplasia. *Cancer* 1983;51:2197–2205.
35. Kojiro M. *Pathology of Hepatocellular Carcinoma.* Oxford, United Kingdom: Blackwell Publishing, 2006.
36. Park YN, Kojiro M, Di Tommaso L, et al. Ductular reaction is helpful in defining early stromal invasion, small hepatocellular carcinomas, and dysplastic nodules. *Cancer* 2007;109:915–923.
37. Kojiro M. Focus on dysplastic nodules and early hepatocellular carcinoma: an Eastern point of view. *Liver Transpl* 2004;10(2 Suppl 1):S3–S8.
38. Takayama T, Makuuchi M, Hirohashi S, et al. Malignant transformation of adenomatous hyperplasia to hepatocellular carcinoma. *Lancet* 1990;336:1150–1153.
39. Kaji K, Terada T, Nakanuma Y. Frequent occurrence of hepatocellular carcinoma in cirrhotic livers after surgical resection of atypical adenomatous hyperplasia (borderline hepatocellular lesion): a follow-up study. *Am J Gastroenterol* 1994;89:903–908.
40. Lencioni R, Caramella D, Bartolozzi C, et al. Percutaneous ethanol injection therapy of adenomatous hyperplastic nodules in cirrhotic liver disease. *Acta Radiol* 1994;35:138–142.
41. Liang P, Dong B, Yu X, et al. Sonography-guided percutaneous microwave ablation of high-grade dysplastic nodules in cirrhotic liver. *AJR Am J Roentgenol* 2005;184:1657–1660.
42. Edmondson HA, Henderson B, Benton B. Liver cell adenomas associated with use of oral contraceptives. *N Engl J Med* 1976;294:470–472.
43. Heinemann LA, Weimann A, Gerken G, et al. Modern oral contraceptive use and benign liver tumors: the German benign liver tumor case-control study. *Eur J Contracept Reprod Health Care* 1998;13:194–200.

44. Bagia S, Hewitt PM, Morris DL. Anabolic steroid-induced hepatic adenomas with spontaneous haemorrhage in a bodybuilder. *Aust N Z J Surg* 2000;70:686–687.

45. Dokmak S, Paradis V, Vilgrain V, et al. A single-center surgical experience of 122 patients with single and multiple hepatocellular adenomas. *Gastroenterology* 2009;137:1698–1705.

46. Welch TJ, Patrick FS, Johnson CM, et al. Focal nodular hyperplasia and hepatic adenoma: comparison of angiography, US, CT and scintigraphy. *Radiology* 1985;156:593–595.

47. Ruppert-Kohlmayr AJ, Uggowitzer MM, Kugler C, et al. Focal nodular hyperplasia and hepatocellular adenoma of the liver: differentiation with multiphasic helical CT. *AJR Am J Roentgenol* 2001;176:1493–1498.

48. Buell JF, Tranchart H, Cannon R, et al. Management of benign hepatic tumors. *Surg Clin N Am* 2010;90:719–735.

49. Reimer P, Tombach B. Hepatic MRI with SPIO: detection and characterization of focal liver lesions. *Eur Radiol* 1998;8:1198–1204.

50. Di Stasi M, Caturelli E, De Sio I, et al. Natural history of focal nodular hyperplasia of the liver: an ultrasound study. *J Clin Ultrasound* 1996;24:345–350.

51. van der Windt DJ, Kok NF, Hussain SM, et al. Case oriented approach to the management of hepatocellular adenoma. *Br J Surg* 2006;93:1495–1502.

52. Karhunen PJ. Benign hepatic tumours and tumour like conditions in men. *J Clin Pathol* 1986;39:183–188.

53. Mortele KJ, Praet M, Van Vlierberghe H, et al. CT and MR imaging findings in focal nodular hyperplasia of the liver: radiologic-pathologic correlation. *AJR Am J Roentgenol* 2000;175:687–692.

54. Bioulac-Sage P, Balabaud C, Wanless IR. Diagnosis of focal nodular hyperplasia: not so easy. *Am J Surg Pathol* 2001;25:1322–1325.

55. Wanless IR, Mawdsley C, Adams R. On the pathogenesis of focal nodular hyperplasia of the liver. *Hepatology* 1985;5:1194–1200.

56. Pain JA, Gimson AE, Williams R, et al. Focal nodular hyperplasia of the liver: results of treatment and options in management. *Gut* 1991;32:524–527.

57. Koffron A, Geller D, Gamblin TC, et al. Laparoscopic liver surgery: shifting the management of liver tumors. *Hepatology* 2006;44:1694–1700.

Genetics and Molecular Biology

■ Introduction

■ Hepatocarcinogenesis is thought to arise through the stepwise accumulation of genetic aberrations resulting from hepatocyte injury and inflammation, often in the context of cirrhosis.[1]

  ● Viral and autoimmune hepatitis, excess alcohol consumption, nonalcoholic fatty liver disease, and inherited metabolic disorders such as hemochromatosis and α-1-antitrypsin deficiency can all cause cirrhosis.

■ Up to 20% of hepatocellular carcinoma (HCC) cases develop in patients without cirrhosis.[2]

  ● Hepatitis B virus (HBV)–induced hepatocarcinogenesis may occur through direct genomic disruption as a result of viral DNA insertion (i.e., insertional mutagenesis).[3]

  ● HCC has been reported in noncirrhotic patients with hereditary hemochromatosis with and without iron overload.[4,5] The initial presence of iron overload may incur damage that persists despite phlebotomy,[5,6] or the C282Y HFE gene mutation itself may be a predisposing factor that can potentiate the damage caused by viral hepatitis and alcohol.[6,7]

  ● In patients with α-1-antitrypsin deficiency who do not have cirrhosis, HCC may develop as a result of intracellular α-1-antitrypsin accumulation, which may be potentially carcinogenic.[8]

■ Some patients develop HCC in the absence of any of these known risk factors.

  ● In a retrospective series of 80 patients who developed HCC in the context of minimal or no background liver fibrosis, only 30 were found to have an identifiable risk factor.[9]

- The patients without any risk factors tended to be younger, and there was no male predominance.[9]

- The male predominance of typical HCC has been observed across multiple series involving both Western and Asian populations. Although this may be partially due to the differential effects of sex hormones on the tumor micro- and macroenvironment,[10] there are also underlying genetic distinctions.

  - Testosterone promotes hepatocarcinogenesis through androgen receptor signal transduction. CAG repeat polymorphisms in exon 1 of the androgen receptor gene affect function; longer repeats are associated with decreased activation of androgen-responsive genes,[11] whereas shorter ($\leq$ 20) repeats appear to increase HCC risk in male HBV carriers.[12]

  - Conversely, in women, the presence of longer ($\geq$ 23) androgen receptor CAG repeats has been associated with an increased risk of HCC.[13]

■ The Molecular Evolution of HCC

- The progressive accumulation and interplay of genetic and molecular alterations drives the evolution of an otherwise normal response to liver injury into a pathogenic process, with the subsequent formation of preneoplastic and neoplastic lesions.[14–16]

  - The preneoplastic phase encompasses the transition of liver inflammation and cirrhosis into dysplastic nodules. Overexpression of the transforming growth factor (*TGF*)-α and insulin-like growth factor (*IGF*)-2 oncogenes promote hepatocyte proliferation. Epigenetic alterations in gene expression and defects in DNA mismatch repair are acquired during this phase. Overexpression of the human telomerase reverse transcriptase (*hTERT*) oncogene and loss of the retinoblastoma 1 (*Rb1*) tumor suppressor also occur.

  - Dysplastic nodules evolve into early HCC with the loss of the *IGF*-2 receptor (*IGF*-2R) oncogene and the tumor suppressors p53, *PTEN*, and *p16*.

- Abnormal expression or activity of the Wnt/β-catenin, epidermal growth factor receptor (EGFR), HGF/c-MET, PI3K, and proangiogenic pathways generates an increasingly malignant phenotype characterized by autonomous tumor growth, survival, and metastasis.
- Genomic structural abnormalities (e.g., loss of heterozygosity, p53 mutations, and chromosomal segment gains and losses) accumulate and diverge as tumors progress from small and well differentiated to large and poorly differentiated.[15]
- Many of these key oncogenes and tumor suppressors are currently being evaluated as therapeutic targets.

■ Oncogenes in HCC

The following described oncogenes are illustrated in **Figure 6.1**.

Epidermal Growth Factor Ligands and Receptors

- EGFR
  - This is a 170-kd protein belonging to the ERBB receptor tyrosine kinase superfamily. It contains extracellular, transmembrane, and intracellular tyrosine.[17]
  - Ligand binding to EGFR leads to receptor dimerization and phosphorylation of downstream effectors, which activate transcription of genes involved in cell growth, proliferation, and survival.[17]
  - EGFR is amplified in up to 70% of HCC tumors, but mutations only occur in < 1% of tumors.[18,19]
- The insulin/IGF-1/IGF-1 receptor (IGF-1R) axis
  - Obesity and the metabolic syndrome lead to hyperinsulinemia, increases in IGF-1, a proinflammatory state that promotes carcinogenesis and are also associated with poorer clinical outcomes.[20]
  - IGF-1R binding by insulin or other steroid hormones activates the PI3K/Akt/mTOR pathway, a key regulator of cell growth, proliferation, survival, and angiogenesis.[21]
  - The insulin/IGF-1R axis also cross-communicates with the EGFR, Her2/neu, and vascular endothelial growth factor receptor (VEGFR) signaling pathways.[22–24]

- IGF-1R upregulation and overexpression have been found in approximately 30–50% of HCC tumors.[22]
- In vitro studies of IGF-1R inhibitors have demonstrated antitumor activity,[22] and clinical trials are ongoing.

▨ Hepatocyte growth factor (HGF) and c-MET receptor
- c-MET is a receptor tyrosine kinase that is activated when bound by its cognate ligand HGF.
- HGF/c-MET activity regulates stromal/mesenchymal interactions that are key for normal organogenesis and tissue regeneration.[25]
- c-MET overexpression has been found in 20–50% of HCC tumors. HBV DNA insertional mutagenesis is one proposed mechanism by which this may occur.[26]
- Data are conflicting with respect to the relationship between c-MET expression, tumor histopathologic features, and survival outcomes.[27,28]
- HGF/c-MET targeting strategies in vitro, including gene therapy and the use of multitargeted tyrosine kinase inhibitors, have shown antitumor activity.[29–31]
- c-MET receptor antagonists in HCC are currently being investigated in clinical trials.

The Wnt/Beta-Catenin Pathway

▨ Wnt/β-catenin signaling controls lineage specification, pattern development, and morphogenesis of developing organisms. It also contributes to liver regeneration.

▨ Secreted Wnt ligands bind to the Frizzled (FRZ) family of cell surface receptors, activating Dishevelled (DSH) intracellular proteins, which, in turn, activate β-catenin. Wnt signaling also conserves β-catenin activity by inhibiting the Axin/GSK-3/APC complex, which normally leads to β-catenin proteolysis.[32]

▨ Activated β-catenin translocates from the cytoplasm to nucleus, activating the transcription of genes promoting cell proliferation and survival, angiogenesis, and extracellular matrix formation.[32]

▨ Dysfunctional pathway activation may occur through activating β-catenin mutations or Axin1 inactivating mutations, which occur in up to 40%[33] and 10% of HCC tumors,[34] each resulting in different tumor phenotypes.[35]

▨ No Wnt/β-catenin targeting agents have been investigated clinically so far.

Angiogenesis

▨ HCC cells rely on a vascular network in order to access the oxygen supply, nutrients, and growth factors necessary for growth and survival.

▨ Angiogenesis is mediated by several factors that affect endothelial cells and the surrounding stroma to promote neovascularization in HCC.

- Angiopoietins bind the Tie-2 receptor tyrosine kinase family and mediate endothelial cell migration, tubule formation, and vessel permeability, but do not have a direct mitogenic effect.[36,37]
- Vascular endothelial growth factors (VEGFs) are dimeric glycoproteins that bind to the VEGFR family of receptor tyrosine kinases and promote endothelial cell growth and survival by activating the PI3K/Akt cascade as well as antiapoptotic signals.[36]
- Platelet-derived growth factor (PDGF), basic fibroblast growth factor (bFGF), and their cognate receptors are other mediators of angiogenesis implicated in HCC.[36,38]

▨ Current agents being used to target the VEGF pathway in HCC do so by one of the following two major mechanisms:

- Monoclonal antibody binding of VEGF to prevent binding to VEGFR (e.g., bevacizumab)
- Multitargeted tyrosine kinase inhibitors (e.g., sorafenib)

Intracellular Signaling Cascades

▨ Ras/Raf/Mek/Erk pathway

- This is a ubiquitous signaling cascade that normally regulates cell growth and survival. Its dysregulation results in autonomous cell growth, proliferation, metastasis, and immortality.[1,39,40]
- Ras and Raf mutations only occur in about 3–4% of HCC tumors.[19] Occupational exposures such as vinyl chloride have been associated with K-ras-2 mutagenesis.[41]

- Strategies to target this pathway that are currently under investigation include:
  - Direct inhibition of Mek1/2
  - Farnesyltransferase inhibition: Functional Ras requires the addition of a farnesyl moiety at its carboxy terminus.[42] 3-hydroxy-3-methyl-glutaryl-coenzyme A (HMG-CoA) reductase inhibitors prevent farnesyl production[43] and are being tested in HCC. Direct farnesyltransferase inhibitors have also been developed.
- PI3K/Akt/mTOR pathway
  - This is another important and ubiquitous signaling cascade that integrates signals from several mitogens including epidermal growth factor (EGF), IGF, and VEGF to promote cell growth, proliferation, and survival.[1,31,44,45]
  - Mammalian target of rapamycin (mTOR) dysregulation has been identified in up to 50% of HCC tumors[44] and appears to be associated with a poor prognosis.[45,46]

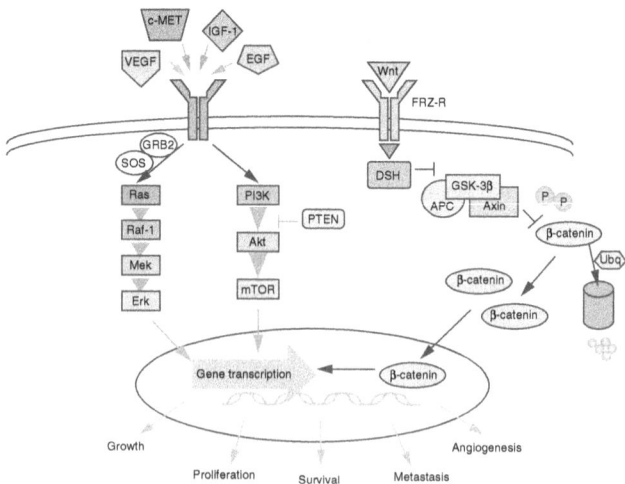

Figure 6.1 Oncogenes and Signaling Pathways Implicated in Hepatocellular Cancer

P, phosphate; Ubq, ubiquitination.

- Patients who have undergone liver transplantation for HCC have been observed to survive longer if given a sirolimus-containing immunosuppressive regimen.[47–50]
- Clinical trials of mTOR inhibition in HCC are ongoing.

■ Tumor Suppressor Genes in HCC

- *TP53*
  - *TP53* plays a vital role in maintaining genomic integrity by regulating the cell cycle, stimulating cell repair mechanisms in response to genomic stress, and promoting apoptosis.[51]
  - Somatic mutations in *TP53* have been identified in 30% of HCC tumors.[19]
    - In endemic areas, mutations occur in > 50% of cases. This is typically caused by aflatoxin B1 exposure, which is associated with a specific G→T transversion at codon 249.[52,53]
    - *TP53*-mutated HCC has poor histopathologic features and prognosis.[54–56]
  - *TP53* may also be inactivated by HBV X viral proteins.[57,58]
- Phosphatase and tensin homolog (*PTEN*)
  - The *PTEN* tumor suppressor gene negatively regulates the PI3K/Akt/mTOR pathway.[56]
  - Normal *PTEN* function may be disrupted by loss of heterozygosity on chromosome 10q23 or by inactivating mutations.[59–61]
  - *PTEN* mutations are found in approximately 5% of HCC tumors.[4]
    - These mutations are associated with genomic instability and may coexist with mutations in *TP53*.[60,62]
- *CDKN2A/p16INK4A*
  - Cyclin-dependent kinase inhibitor 2A is encoded by the *p16* gene on chromosome 9p21–22. It is an important cell cycle checkpoint regulator at the junction between G_1 and S phase. *CDKN2A* binds cyclin-dependent kinase 4 (CDK4), preventing its interaction with cyclin D, which is necessary for cell cycle progression.[63]
  - *p16* gene alterations (point mutations, promoter hypermethylation, and homozygous deletions) have been

reported in up to 70% of HCC tumors, suggesting a potential role in hepatocarcinogenesis.[64]

- Mutations of *CDKN2A* have been associated with a poor prognosis in recurrent early stage HCC.[62]

MicroRNA in HCC

- MicroRNAs are highly conserved, short, noncoding nucleotide sequences that regulate gene expression. They were first described as key molecules that orchestrate the timing and sequencing of larval development in the *Caenorhabditis elegans* worm.[65]
- MicroRNAs also have a role in regulating cell growth, survival, and apoptosis; immune and stress responses; metabolism; and tumorigenesis.[65]
- In cancer, microRNAs exhibit distinct tumor specificity and have been shown to have pathogenic and prognostic relevance in HCC.[66]
  - miR-26 expression has been shown to be differentially expressed in men and women. Patients with low levels of miR-26 expression had a poorer prognosis but responded better to interferon.[67]
- MicroRNAs may contribute to the survival of HCC stem cells, leading to disease recurrences. Thus, microRNA may serve as potential therapeutic target.
  - EpCAM-positive hepatic cancer stem cells express high levels of miR-181. In in-vitro studies, miR-181 inhibition has been shown to reduce stem cell tumorigenicity and spheroid colony formation.[68]

Virus–Tumor Molecular Interactions

- Liver damage caused by the various hepatotoxins and carcinogens may be potentiated by a concurrent viral hepatitis infection and vice versa.
- Asian male carriers of HBV who have androgen receptors with short CAG repeats have a higher risk of developing HCC compared to those with short repeats.[12] Female HBV carriers who have androgen receptors with long CAG repeats appear to have a significantly higher risk of HCC and tend to develop it at a younger age than

noncarriers. In younger women, hepatocarcinogenesis may be promoted through these altered receptors as a result of binding to estrogen in the presence of specific co-activators.[13]

▨ Different effectors of the Wnt/β-catenin pathway are mutated depending on the type of viral hepatitis infection. The presence of a hepatitis C virus (HCV) infection appears to be associated with β-catenin mutations,[32] whereas HBV infection has been associated with Axin1 mutations.[69]

▨ Infection with HCV can instigate aberrant pathway activity by upregulating Raf1. This may explain why HCV-infected patients appear to be more sensitive to sorafenib compared to those with other causes of liver disease.[70–72]

▨ HBV and HCV infections have been associated with different chromosomal structural changes.[73,74]

■ Molecular Subtypes of HCC

▨ Global gene expression profiling has identified subtypes of HCC that may provide information on the cell of origin and that also have prognostic relevance.

▨ HB and HC subtypes refer to HCCs derived from hepatoblasts and hepatocytes, respectively. The HB subtype has been shown to be independently associated with disease recurrence and worse survival. This may be due to the expression of the *MMP1, PLAUR, TIMP1, CD44,* and *VIL2* genes, which mediate the degradation of tissue barriers and facilitate invasion and metastasis.[75]

▨ The HB and HC subtypes can also be stratified into clusters A and B. Cluster A HCCs demonstrate increased cell proliferation and antiapoptotic gene expression. Genes involved in ubiquitination and sumoylation, which lead to the degradation of tumor suppressors and other growth-inhibiting molecules, are also overexpressed. The poorer prognosis of cluster A HCCs compared with cluster B HCCs is consistent with this profile.[76]

▨ It should be noted that these clusters are not discrete entities and that considerable overlap occurs.[73,74] In addition, these preliminary subtypes require further investigation and validation before they can be used clinically.

- MicroRNAs can also identify HCC subclasses characterized by distinct genetic signatures and phenotypes that may potentially be used to guide therapy.[77]

Fibrolamellar HCC (FLL-HCC)

- The molecular and genetic origins of this rare variant of HCC (see Chapter 1) are mostly unknown. Small studies have identified several molecular and genetic aberrations.
- FLL-HCC appears to be more genetically stable than typical HCC.[78] Mutations in TP53 and b-catenin, often found in typical HCC, are uncommon in FLL-HCC.[79–81]
- Epigenetic modulation (e.g., methylation) of tumor suppressors appears to be a rare event in FLL-HCC. Gene methylation levels are similar to those found in normal liver parenchyma as well as HCC arising from nonviral cirrhosis.[82]
- Common sites of chromosomal aberrations in FLL-HCC include gains of 1q, 7p, 7q, 8q and loss of 18q.[78,84] A gain of 1q potentially implicates the *PI3K/Akt/mTOR* pathway.[78] Gains of 7p and 7q involve the *EGFR* and *HGF/c-MET* oncogenes, respectively. Loss of 18q implicates the deleted in colon cancer (*DCC*), deleted in pancreatic cancer locus 4 (*DPC4*) and S*mad4* tumor suppressors.[78,83] These changes are associated with more aggressive behavior and occur at a higher frequency in metastatic and recurrent FLL-HCC than in primary tumors. Similar chromosomal aberrations are also found in advanced typical HCC.[83]
- Overexpression of aromatase,[84] Ras, mitogen-activated protein kinase (MAPK), and lipid and protein metabolism pathways has also been identified in FLL-HCC and may be involved in its pathogenesis.[85,86]

■ References

1. Whittaker S, Marais R, Zhu AX. The role of signaling pathways in the development and treatment of hepatocellular carcinoma. *Oncogene* 2010;29:4989–5005.
2. Nzeako UC, Goodman ZD, Ishak KG. Hepatocellular carcinoma in cirrhotic and non cirrhotic livers. A clinico-histopathologic study of 804 North American patients. *Am J Clin Pathol* 1996;105:65–75.

3. Cougot D, Neuveut C, Buendia MA. HBV induced carcinogenesis. *J Clin Virol* 2005;34(Suppl 1):S75–S78.

4. Singh P, Kaur H, Lerner RG, et al. Hepatocellular carcinoma in non-cirrhotic liver without evidence of iron overload in a patient with primary hemochromatosis. Review. *J Gastrointest Oncol* [Epub ahead of print on September 28, 2010].

5. Grando-Lemaire V, Guettier C, Chevret S, et al. Hepatocellular carcinoma without cirrhosis in the West: epidemiological factors and histopathology of the non-tumorous liver. *J Hepatol* 1999;31:508–513.

6. Hiatt T, Trotter JF, Kam I. Hepatocellular carcinoma in a noncirrhotic patient with hereditary hemochromatosis. *Am J Med Sci* 2007;334:228–230.

7. Fargion S, Stazi MA, Fracanzani AL, et al. Mutations in the HFE gene and their interaction with exogenous risk factors in hepatocellular carcinoma. *Blood Cells Mol Dis* 2001;27: 505–511.

8. Zhou H, Fischer HP. Liver carcinoma in PiZ alpha-1-antitrypsin deficiency. *Am J Surg Pathol* 1998;22:742–748.

9. Bralet MP, Regimbeau JM, Pineau P, et al. Hepatocellular carcinoma occurring in nonfibrotic liver: epidemiologic and histopathologic analysis of 80 French cases. *Hepatology* 2000;32:200–204.

10. Yeh SH, Chen PJ. Gender disparity in hepatocellular carcinoma: the roles of sex hormones. *Oncology* 2010;78(Suppl 1):172–179.

11. Chamberlain NL, Driver ED, Miesfeld RL. The length and location of CAG trinucleotide repeats in the androgen receptor N-terminal domain affect transactivation function. *Nucleic Acids Res* 1994;22:3181–3186.

12. Yu MW, Cheng SW, Lin MW, et al. Androgen-receptor gene CAG repeats, plasma testosterone levels, and risk of hepatitis B-related hepatocellular carcinoma. *J Natl Cancer Inst* 2000;92:2023–2028.

13. Yu MW, Yang YC, Yang SY, et al. Androgen receptor exon 1 CAG repeat length and risk of hepatocellular carcinoma in women. *Hepatology* 2002;36:156–163.

14. Whittaker S, Marais R, Zhu AX. The role of signaling pathways in the development and treatment of hepatocellular carcinoma. *Oncogene* 2010;29:4989–5005.

15. Thorgeirsson SS, Grisham JW. Molecular pathogenesis of human hepatocellular carcinoma. *Nat Genet* 2002;31: 339–346.

16. Grisham JW. Molecular genetic alterations in primary hepatocellular neoplasms: hepatocellular adenoma, hepatocellular carcinoma, and hepatoblastoma. In: Coleman WB, Tsongalis GJ (eds). *The Molecular Basis of Human Cancer*. Totowa, NJ: Humana Press, 2001:269–346.

17.   Schlessinger J. Ligand-induced, receptor-mediated dimerization and activation of EGF receptor. *Cell* 2002;110:669–672.

18.   Ito Y, Takeda T, Sakon M, et al. Expression and clinical significance of erb-B receptor family in hepatocellular carcinoma. *Br J Cancer* 2001;84:1377–1383.

19.   Wellcome Trust Genome Campus, Sanger Institute.
Catalogue of Somatic Mutations in Cancer (COSMIC) database. 2008. http://www.sanger.ac.uk/genetics/CGP/cosmic/.

20.   Hursting SD, Berger NA. Energy balance, host-related factors,
and cancer progression. *J Clin Oncol* 2010;28:4058–4065.

21.   Pollak M. Insulin and insulin-like growth factor signalling
in neoplasia. *Nat Rev Cancer* 2008;8:915–928 [Erratum in:
Nat Rev Cancer 2009;9:224].

22.   Desbois-Mouthon C, Baron A, Blivet-Van Eggelpoël MJ,
et al. Insulin-like growth factor-1 receptor inhibition induces a resistance mechanism via the epidermal growth
factor receptor/HER3/AKT signaling pathway: rational basis
for cotargeting insulin-like growth factor-1 receptor and epidermal growth factor receptor in hepatocellular carcinoma.
Clin Cancer Res 2009;15:5445–5456.

23.   Lu Y, Zi X, Zhao Y, et al. Insulin-like growth factor-I receptor
signaling and resistance to trastuzumab (Herceptin). *J Natl
Cancer Inst* 2001;93:1852–1857.

24.   Slomiany MG, Black LA, Kibbey MM, et al. IGF-1 induced
vascular endothelial growth factor secretion in head and neck
squamous cell carcinoma. *Biochem Biophys Res Commun*
2006;342:851–858.

25.   Matsomoto K, Nakamura T. Emerging multipotent aspects
of hepatocyte growth factor. *J Biochem* 1996;119:591–600.

26.   Tiollais P, Hsu TY, Moroy T, et al. Hepadnavirus as an inser-
tional mutagen in hepatocellular carcinoma. In: Hollinger
FB, Lemon SM, Margolis HS (eds). *Viral Hepatitis and Liver
Disease.* Baltimore: Williams & Wilkins, 1990:541–546.

27.   Kaposi-Novak P, Lee JS, Gomez-Quiroz L, et al. Met-regulated
expression signature defines a subset of human hepatocellular carcinomas with poor prognosis and aggressive phenotype.
J Clin Invest 2006;116:1582–1595.

28.   Huitzil FD, Sun MY, Capanu M, et al. Expression of the c-
met and HGF in resected hepatocellular carcinoma (rHCC):
correlation with clinicopathological features (CP) and overall
survival (OS) [abstract]. *J Clin Oncol* 2008;26(Suppl):4599.

29.   Salvi A, Arici B, Portolani N, et al. In vitro c-met inhibition by antisense RNA and plasmid-based RNAi down-
modulates migration and invasion of hepatocellular carcinoma cells. *Int J Oncol* 2007;31:451–460.

30.   Heideman DA, Overmeer RM, van Beusechem VW, et al.
Inhibition of angiogenesis and HGF-cMET-elicited malignant processes in human hepatocellular carcinoma cells

using adenoviral vector-mediated NK4 gene therapy. *Cancer Gene Ther* 2005;12:954–962.

31. Wang R, Ferrell LD, Faouzi S, et al. Activation of the Met receptor by cell attachment induces and sustains hepatocellular carcinomas in transgenic mice. *J Cell Biol* 2001;153:1023–1034.

32. Avila MA, Berasain C, Sangro B, et al. New therapies for hepatocellular carcinoma. *Oncogene* 2006;25:3866–3884.

33. Huang H, Fujii H, Sankila A, et al. Beta-catenin mutations are frequent in human hepatocellular carcinomas associated with hepatitis C virus infection. *Am J Pathol* 1999;155:1795–1801.

34. Taniguchi K, Roberts LR, Aderca IN, et al. Mutational spectrum of beta-catenin, ASCIN 1 and AXIN2 in hepatocellular carcinomas and hepatoblastomas. *Oncogene* 2002;21:4863–4871.

35. Cieply B, Zeng G, Proverbs-Singh T, et al. Unique phenotype of hepatocellular cancers with exon-3 mutations in beta-catenin gene. *Hepatology* 2009;49:821–831.

36. Sturk C, Dumont D. Angiogenesis. In: Tannock IF, Hill R, Bristow R, et al (eds). *Basic Science of Oncology*. Toronto: McGraw-Hill Medical Publishing Division, 2005:231–248.

37. Mitsuhashi N, Shimizu H, Ohtsuka M, et al. Angiopoietins and Tie-2 expression in angiogenesis and proliferation of human hepatocellular carcinoma. *Hepatology* 2003;37:1105–1113.

38. Zhang T, Sun HC, Xu Y, et al. Overexpression of platelet-derived growth factor receptor alpha in endothelial cells of hepatocellular carcinoma associated with high metastatic potential. *Clin Cancer Res* 2005;11:8557–8563.

39. Gollob JA, Wilhelm S, Carter C, et al. Role of Raf kinase in cancer: therapeutic potential of targeting the Raf/MEK/ERK signal transduction pathway. *Semin Oncol* 2006;33:392–406.

40. Hwang YH, Choi JY, Kim S, et al. Over-expression of c-raf-1 proto-oncogene in liver cirrhosis and hepatocellular carcinoma. *Hepatol Res* 2004;29:113–121.

41. Weihrauch M, Benick M, Lehner G, et al. High prevalence of K-ras-2 mutations in hepatocellular carcinomas in workers exposed to vinyl chloride. *Int Arch Occup Environ Health* 2001;74:405–410.

42. Kato K, Cox AD, Hisaka MM, et al. Isoprenoid addition to Ras protein is the critical modification for its membrane association and transforming activity. *Proc Natl Acad Sci USA* 1992;89:6403–6407.

43. Goldstein JL, Brown MS. Regulation of the mevalonate pathway. *Nature* 1990;343:425–430.

44. Treiber G. mTOR inhibitors for hepatocellular cancer: a forward-moving target. *Expert Rev Anticancer Ther* 2009;9: 247–261.

45. Villanueva A, Chiang DY, Newell P, et al. Pivotal role of mTOR signaling in hepatocellular carcinoma. *Gastroenterology* 2007; 135:1972–1983.

46. Baba H, Wohlschlaeger J, Cicinnati VR, et al. Phosphorylation of p70S6 kinase predicts survival in patients with clear-margin resected hepatocellular carcinoma. *Liver Int* 2009;29:399–405.
47. Chen YB, Sun YA, Gong JP. Effects of rapamycin in liver transplantation. *Hepatobiliary Pancreas Dis Int* 2008;7:25–28.
48. Toso S, Merani S, Bigam DL, et al. Sirolimus-based immunosuppression is associated with increased survival after liver transplantation for hepatocellular carcinoma. *Hepatology* 2010; 51:1237–1243.
49. Zhou J, Fan J, Wang Z, et al. Conversion to sirolimus immunosuppression in liver transplantation recipients with hepatocellular carcinoma: report of an initial experience. *World J Gastroenterol* 2006;12:3114–3118.
50. Zimmerman MA, Trotter JF, Wachs M, et al. Sirolimus-based immunosuppression following liver transplantation for hepatocellular carcinoma. *Liver Transpl* 2008;14:633–638.
51. Oster S, Penn L, Stambolic V. Oncogenes and tumor suppressor genes. In: Tannock IF, Hill R, Bristow R, et al (eds). *Basic Science of Oncology*. Toronto: McGraw-Hill Medical Publishing Division, 2005:123–141.
52. Bressac B, Kew M, Wands J, et al. Selective G to T mutations of p53 in hepatocellular carcinoma from southern Africa. *Nature* 1991;350:429–431.
53. Hsu IC, Metcalf RA, Sun T, et al. Mutational hotspot in the p53 gene in human hepatocellular carcinomas. *Nature* 1991;350:427–428.
54. Hayashi H, Sugio K, Matsumata T, et al. The clinical significance of p53 gene mutation in hepatocellular carcinomas from Japan. *Hepatology* 1995;22:1702–1707.
55. Honda K, Sbisa E, Tullo A, et al. P53 mutation is a poor prognostic indicator for survival in patients with hepatocellular carcinoma undergoing surgical tumour ablation. *Br J Cancer* 1998;77:776–782.
56. Stambolic V, Suzuk A, de la Pompa JL, et al. Negative regulation of PKB/Akt-dependent cell survival by the tumor suppressor PTEN. *Cell* 1998;95:29–39.
57. Wang XW, Forrester K, Yeh H, et al. Hepatitis B virus X protein inhibits p53 sequence-specific DNA binding, transcriptional activity and association with transcription factor ERCC3. *Proc Natl Acad Sci USA* 1994;91:2230–2234.
58. Truant R, Antunovic J, Greenblatt J, et al. Direct interaction of the hepatitis B virus HBX protein with p53 leads to inhibition by HBX of p53 response element-directed transactivation. *J Virol* 1995;69:1851–1859.
59. Bae JJ, Rho JW, Lee TJ, et al. Loss of heterozygosity on chromosome 10q23 and mutation of the phosphatase tensin homolog deleted from chromosome 10 tumors suppressor

gene in Korean hepatocellular carcinoma patients. *Oncol Rep* 2007;18:1007–1013.

60. Yao YJ, Ping XL, Zhang H, et al. PTEN/MMAC1 mutations in hepatocellular carcinomas. *Oncogene* 1999;18:3181–3185.

61. Kawamura N, Nagai H, Bando K, et al. PTEN/MMAC1 mutations in hepatocellular carcinomas: somatic inactivation of both alleles in tumors. *Jpn J Cancer Res* 1999;90:413–418.

62. Imbeaud S, Ladeiro Y, Zucman-Rossi J. Identification of novel oncogenes and tumor suppressors in hepatocellular carcinoma. *Semin Liver Dis* 2001;30:75–86.

63. Serrano M, Hannon GJ, Neach D. A new regulatory motif in cell-cycle control causing specific inhibition of cyclin D/CDK4. *Nature* 1993;366:704–707.

64. Liew CT, Li HM, Lo KW, et al. High frequency of p16INK4A gene alterations in hepatocellular carcinoma. *Oncogene* 1999;18:789–795.

65. Reinhart BJ, Slack FJ, Basson M, et al. The 21-nucleotide let-7 RNA regulates developmental timing in *Caenorhabditis elegans*. *Nature* 2000;403:901–906.

66. Ji J, Wang XW. New kids on the block: diagnostic and prognostic microRNAs in hepatocellular carcinoma. *Cancer Biol Ther* 2009;8:1686–1693.

67. Ji J, Shi J, Budhu A, et al. MicroRNA expression, survival, and response to interferon in liver cancer. *N Engl J Med* 2009;361:1437–1447.

68. Ji J, Yamashita T, Budhu A, et al. Identification of microRNA-181 by genome-wide screening as a critical player in EpCAM-positive hepatic cancer stem cells. *Hepatology* 2009;50:472–480.

69. Laurent-Puig P, Legoix P, Bluteau O, et al. Genetic alterations associated with hepatocellular carcinomas define distinct pathways of hepatocarcinogenesis. *Gastroenterology* 2001;120:1763–1773.

70. Huitzil FD, Saltz LS, Song J, et al. Retrospective analysis of outcome in hepatocellular carcinoma (HCC) patients (pts) with hepatitis C (C+) versus B (B+) treated with sorafenib (S). Program and Abstracts of the 2008 Gastrointestinal Cancers Symposium, January 19–21, 2008, Orlando, FL, Abstract 173.

71. Bolondi L, Caspary W, Bennouna J, et al. Clinical benefit of sorafenib in hepatitis C patients with hepatocellular carcinoma (HCC): subgroup analysis of the SHARP trial. 2008 Gastrointestinal Cancers Symposium, Orlando, FL, Abstract 129.

72. Giambartolomei S, Covone F, Levrero M, et al. Sustained activation of the Raf/MEK/Erk pathway in response to EGF in stable cell lines expressing the hepatitis C virus (HCV) core protein. *Oncogene* 2001;20:2606–2610.

73. Wong N, Lai P, Pang E, et al. Genomic aberrations in human hepatocellular carcinomas of differing etiologies. *Clin Cancer Res* 2000;6:4000–4009.

74. Marchio A, Pineau P, Meddeb M, et al. Distinct chromosomal abnormality pattern in primary liver cancer of non-B, non-C patients. *Oncogene* 2000;19:3733–3738.

75. Lee JS, Heo J, Libbrecht L, et al. A novel prognostic subtype of human hepatocellular carcinoma derived from hepatic progenitor cells. *Nat Med* 2006;12:410–416.

76. Lee JS, Thorgeirsson SS. Genome-scale profiling of gene expression in hepatocellular carcinoma: classification, survival prediction, and identification of therapeutic targets. *Gastroenterology* 2004;127:S51–S55.

77. Toffanin S, Hoshida J, Lachenmayer A, et al. MicroRNA-based classification of hepatocellular carcinoma and oncogenic role of miR-517a. *Gastroenterology* 2011;140: 1618–1628.

78. Ward SC, Waxman S. Fibrolamellar carcinoma: a review with focus on genetics and comparison to other malignant primary liver tumors. Semin Liver Dis 2011 Feb;31(1):61–70

79. Kannangai R, Wang J, Liu QZ, et al. Survivin overexpression in hepatocellular carcinoma is associated with p53 dysregulation. *Int J Gastrointest Cancer* 2005;35:53–60.

80. Terris B, Pineau P, Bregeaud L, et al. Close correlation between beta-catenin gene alterations and nuclear accumulation of the protein in human hepatocellular carcinomas. *Oncogene* 1999;18:6583–6588.

81. Wellcome Trust Genome Campus, Sanger Institute. Catalogue of Somatic Mutations in Cancer (COSMIC) database. 2008. http://www.sanger.ac.uk/genetics/CGP/cosmic/.

82. Vivekanandan P, Torbensen M. Epigenetic instability is rare in fibrolamellar carcinomas but high in viral-associated hepatocellular carcinomas. *Mod Pathol* 2008;21:670–675.

83. Kakar S, Chen X, Ho C, et al. Chromosomal changes in fibrolamellar hepatocellular carcinoma detected by array comparative genomic hybridization. *Mod Pathol* 2009;22:134–141.

84. Agarwal VR, Takayama K, Van Wyk JJ, et al. Molecular basis of severe gynecomastia associated with aromatase expression in a fibrolamellar hepatocellular carcinoma. *Clin Endocrinol Metab* 1998;83:1797–1800.

85. Sahin F, Kannangai R, Adgebola O, et al. mTOR and P70 S6 kinase expression in primary liver neoplasms. *Clin Cancer Res* 2004;10:8421–8425.

86. Kannangai R, Vivekanandan P, Martinez-Murillo F, et al. Fibrolamellar carcinomas show overexpression of genes in the RAS, MAPK, PIK3 and xenobiotic degradation pathways. *Hum Pathol* 2007;38:639–644.

CHAPTER 7

Management

■ How Does Underlying Liver Dysfunction Influence Treatment?

The extent of hepatic dysfunction is a key determinant of the prognostic outcome of patients with hepatocellular carcinoma (HCC). It influences a patient's eligibility for treatment, as well as the treatment approach. Patients with disease limited to the liver and not involving the major blood vessels who have adequate liver function are eligible for curative treatments such as surgery or transplantation. Patients with hepatic decompensation are also candidates for transplantation if they have early-stage HCC. Patients with poorer hepatic reserve and more extensive HCC are treated with palliative intent. The Barcelona Clinical Liver Cancer (BCLC)[1] staging and treatment algorithm is an example of how these factors can be synthesized in the decision-making process, but in clinical practice it is often difficult to separate patients into such discrete groups. A recent expert consensus statement acknowledged the heterogeneity among patients with BCLC intermediate- or advanced-stage HCC, stating that some might still be surgical candidates even though the algorithm suggests nonsurgical ablative or systemic therapy.[2] Thus, each case needs to be evaluated individually by a multidisciplinary team.

Surgery

■ For those with preserved liver function and low-volume disease without major vessel involvement (i.e., American Joint Committee on Cancer TNM seventh edition stage I–IIIA), partial hepatectomy offers the best chance for long-term survival and cure.

- Five-year survival rates are typically in range of 40–50%, but rates as high as 78% and 93% have been reported.[3,4]
- The best outcomes are associated with solitary or oligonodular disease, small tumors (diameter ≤ 5 cm), no vascular or capsular invasion, clean margins (≥ 1 cm if possible), Child-Pugh A or, in some instances, B cirrhosis, and the absence of intrahepatic metastases.[3–5]
- Recurrence rates after hepatectomy are high, ranging from 60–100%, and are most commonly due to the development of intrahepatic metastases.[6]

Assessing Resectability

- Medical resectability: In addition to a routine preoperative assessment, several unique considerations are important in evaluation of a patient about to undergo a hepatic resection. These factors help to estimate the risk of perioperative morbidity and mortality.
- The most important determinant of the 30-day postoperative mortality rate (i.e., rate of death occurring within 30 days of surgery) is cirrhosis. This rate ranges from 7–25% for patients with cirrhosis due to the higher risk of postoperative hepatic decompensation compared to < 3% for those without cirrhosis.[7]
- The presence of portal venous hypertension (≥ 10 mm Hg), often manifested by an elevated bilirubin, significantly increases the risk of postoperative decompensation and appears to be more important than Child-Pugh score.[8]
  - The 5-year survival rate for patients with both normal serum bilirubin and portal venous pressure was 70% in one series. This decreased to 50% for those with portal hypertension and to < 30% for those with both portal hypertension and an elevated serum bilirubin.[8]
  - Portal venous pressure is estimated using both clinical findings and diagnostic imaging.
    - Clinical manifestations include thrombocytopenia (< 100/mL), the presence of esophageal varices, ascites, and splenomegaly.[9]
    - The "gold standard" for measuring portal venous pressure is by direct catheterization of the portal

vein. Noninvasive techniques are available such as duplex Doppler ultrasonography.[10]

- Surgical resectability is determined by the extent of disease as seen on imaging studies including triphasic computed tomography (CT) scans or magnetic resonance imaging (MRI) of the abdomen. Although outcomes are better for those with low-volume disease without cirrhosis, the presence of multinodular disease, lesions > 5 cm in diameter, and portal hypertension should not be considered absolute contraindications to hepatectomy; cases should be assessed individually.[2]
  - An estimate of the future liver remnant (FLR) is an important predictor of the safety of surgery and postoperative outcomes.[11]
    - The FLR refers to the volume of liver left behind after hepatectomy.
    - The FLR can be accurately measured preoperatively using CT imaging.[12] In addition, an equation has been developed and validated to calculate the healthy liver volume required for optimal function based on body weight[13]: Liver volume (mL) = 706.2 × body surface area (m^2) + 2.4.
    - An FLR ≤ 25% of the preoperative volume has been associated with a significant increase in postoperative portal hypertension and liver parenchymal injury.[11] However, there is no consensus regarding the absolute FLR cutoff below which resection is considered unsafe.
  - Preoperative portal vein embolization (PVE)
    - PVE occludes a branch of the portal vein to cause ipsilateral hepatic lobe atrophy and compensatory hypertrophy of the contralateral lobe.[14]
    - PVE can improve the success and safety of hepatectomy by inducing hypertrophy of the remnant liver.[11,14] In one series, preoperative PVE increased the FLR from 25% to 80%.[11]

Preoperative Therapy

- The majority of newly diagnosed patients do not have surgically resectable disease at presentation. The use of various preoperative treatments may convert unresectable disease into resectable disease through tumor downstaging.

- Other theoretical benefits of preoperative therapy include a reduction in the risk of recurrence by controlling micrometastases through earlier exposure to systemic therapy. Furthermore, patients whose disease progresses on such therapy can be spared from an unnecessary surgery.
- Locoregional ablative therapies
  - Transarterial embolization of the hepatic artery with or without chemotherapy (see Nonsurgical Locally Ablative Therapies) causes tumor cell death through ischemic and cytotoxic mechanisms.
    - Transarterial chemoembolization (TACE) can convert unresectable disease to resectable disease, and 5-year survival rates of up to 56% have been reported.[15] However, other series have reported either no survival benefit[16,17] or worse outcomes[18,19] with preoperative TACE.
    - Shorter disease-free survival has been observed in patients who demonstrate partial responses to TACE as opposed to complete or no response. It is possible that in partially necrosed tumors, cell-cell adhesions are weakened between viable and dead cells as a result of procedure-related manipulation, facilitating the metastasis of viable tumor cells. In contrast, complete responders would theoretically have no viable cells left and those who did not respond might maintain intact intercellular adhesions.[16]
    - TACE must be used cautiously in cirrhotic patients because the risk of acute hepatic decompensation and bleeding are significantly higher compared to untreated patients.[18,20,21]
    - Combining TACE with PVE has the additive effect of increasing the FLR volume while occluding the tumor blood supply and inducing tumor necrosis.[22,23]
  - Radioembolization (see Nonsurgical Locally Ablative Therapies) occludes a branch of the hepatic artery with radiolabeled beads to selectively irradiate the affected liver segment.

- Radioparticles that have been studied in this setting include yttrium-90 (^{90}Y)-labeled microspheres, iodine-131 (^{131}I)-antiferritin, and ^{131}I-labeled lipiodol. Between 27% and 74% of patients have > 50% reduction in tumor volume, including pathologic complete responses in a quarter of patients.[24–26]
- Systemic therapy such as the combination of cisplatin, interferon-α, doxorubicin, and 5-fluorouracil (the PIAF regimen; see Systemic Therapy) has been evaluated in the preoperative setting with promising results.[27]
  - Eighteen percent of patients had > 50% regression in tumor size, including two complete responses. Ten percent of patients achieved conversion to resectable disease and underwent curative resections. One- and 3-year survival rates were 100% and 53%, respectively. Ten patients had durable remissions after 27 months of follow-up.
  - Treatment was well tolerated overall. However, one patient had reactivation of a prior hepatitis B infection that was successfully treated before surgery.
- There is no standard preferred approach. The various locoregional or systemic therapies alone or in combination are effective at inducing tumor responses and as conversion strategies in patients with unresectable HCC.
  - The vast majority of patients respond to therapy, and complete pathologic responses have been reported in approximately 20–25% of cases.[15,28]
  - Sixty to 100% of patients with initially unresectable HCC are converted to having resectable disease.[15,24,28]
  - Five-year survival rates range from 45–62%.[15,24,28,29]
- The choice of preoperative therapy depends on the clinical picture including the disease extent, patient comorbidities and preferences, and local expertise.

Adjuvant Therapy

- Postoperative recurrences occur in 60–100% of patients and are usually intrahepatic.[6] Risk factors include close (< 10 mm) or positive margins, intravascular invasion, intrahepatic metastases, and absence of tumor encapsulation.[30]

- Adjuvant therapy has not demonstrated any definitive survival benefit thus far; therefore, it is not recommended for routine use. Several approaches have been or are currently under investigation.
- Experience with adjuvant systemic or hepatic intra-arterial chemotherapy in HCC is limited because its activity has primarily been explored in retrospective reviews that have shown conflicting results.[30,31] Recently, adjuvant capecitabine significantly improved time to progression and decreased the risk of recurrence, but had no overall survival benefit compared to surgery alone.[32]
- Lipiodol is a poppy seed oil derivative typically used as an embolic substance in transarterial embolizations. Adjuvant intra-arterial[131] I-labeled lipiodol has been studied in retrospective and prospective studies, both of which report significant decreases in the risk of tumor recurrence along with improved survival outcomes.[33,34]
  - Compared to surgery alone, a single dose of intra-arterial[131] I-labeled lipiodol has been shown to significantly improve disease-free and overall survival up to 7 years after treatment. At 10 years of follow-up, however, the differences were no longer found to be significant. A proposed explanation was the underlying propensity of cirrhotic patients to develop HCC and the inability of treatment to prevent recurrences outside of the radiation field.[33]
- Retinoic acid is a vitamin A derivative that has been shown to activate DNA repair mechanisms or induce apoptosis of hepatoma cells containing carcinogen-DNA adducts.[35]
  - In a prospective adjuvant trial, peretinoin prevented the occurrence of second primary HCC tumors after curative surgery or percutaneous ethanol ablation.[36] Survival at 6 years was 74% versus 46% for the placebo group.[37]
  - A larger phase II/III trial of high- and low-dose peretinoin compared to placebo did not meet the primary end point of significantly improving recurrence-free survival. However, a strong dose–response relationship was observed such that high-dose peretinoin significantly reduced the hazard ratio for recurrence after 2 years.[38]

- Sorafenib is the current first-line standard therapy for advanced HCC (see Systemic Therapy). It is currently being evaluated in the phase III placebo-controlled Sorafenib as Adjuvant Treatment in the Prevention of Recurrence of Hepatocellular Carcinoma (STORM) trial (ClinicalTrials.gov, NCT00692770). Its use in the adjuvant setting is not recommended and will depend on the outcome of the STORM trial.

Orthotopic Liver Transplantation (OLT)

- OLT is a definitive treatment for HCC because it removes the tumor while also replacing the diseased liver parenchyma, making it the preferred treatment modality for patients with multinodular disease and/or more advanced cirrhosis.[2] Given limited resources, stringent criteria have been implemented in order to prioritize candidates in a way that is equitable and medically sound.

Assessing Eligibility and Priority for OLT

- The Milan criteria are well established guidelines. Patients with a solitary lesion ≤ 5 cm in diameter *or* up to three lesions each ≤ 3 cm, no gross vascular invasion, and no lymph node or distant metastases who undergo OLT have a reported 4-year survival rate of 75%.[39]
- Some patients who exceed the Milan criteria can still benefit from OLT. Those who meet the "Up to Seven Rule" (diameter of largest tumor [cm] + number of tumors = 7) for OLT have a reported 5-year survival rate ≥ 70%.[40]
- The University of California San Francisco (UCSF) criteria are even less restrictive; patients with a single nodule < 6.5 cm *or* one to three nodules all ≤ 4.5 cm and a total disease diameter < 8 cm are considered eligible. Survival at 5 years using these criteria was reportedly 75%. Importantly, none of these patients underwent downstaging therapy before OLT.[41]
  - The applicability of the UCSF criteria has been questioned. A retrospective comparison of the UCSF and Milan criteria reported a posttransplantation 5-year survival rate of only 45% for patients who met UCSF

but not Milan criteria, compared with 60% for patients who met both criteria.[42]

■ The "Metroticket Paradigm" pooled data from 35 international transplantation centers of patients who exceed the Milan criteria. Tumor size and number are mapped onto a Cartesian plane such that each dot corresponds to a "city" location. The further away the "city" from the region encompassing the Milan criteria, the higher is the "cost" in terms of the reduction in anticipated 5-year survival after transplantation.[43] A strength of this model is that it is dynamic, and additional factors such as vascular invasion, donor, and dropout rates can be integrated to improve the precision for predicting survival outcomes.[43]

    ● A Metroticket calculator predicting 3- and 5-year survival is available at the following website: http://89.96.76.14/metroticket/calculator/.

■ In the United States, the Model for End-Stage Liver Disease (MELD) score is used to prioritize patients for organ allocation by estimating 3-month mortality risk due to end-stage liver disease (**Table 7.1**). The MELD score is calculated using serum bilirubin, creatinine, and international normalized ratio (INR) and has been validated in patients with various causes of cirrhosis.[44]

    ● MELD = 3.8 [Ln serum bilirubin (mg/dL)] + 11.2 (Ln INR) + 9.6 [Ln serum creatinine (mg/dL)] + 6.4

    ● A MELD calculator is available at the following website: www.mayoclinic.org/MELD.

Table 7.1   The MELD Score for Patients with Advanced Cirrhosis and Associated 3-Month Mortality

MELD Score	3-Month Mortality
> 40	71.3%
30–39	52.6%
20–29	19.6%
10–19	6%
< 9	1.9%

■ Given the concern that many transplantation candidates might progress and/or decompensate while waiting, the United Network for Organ Sharing (UNOS) developed an additional prioritization scheme using the American Liver Tumor Study Group (ALTSG) modification of the tumor, node, metastasis (TNM) staging system. Patients with stage II disease (single nodule 2–5 cm or two to three nodules all ≤ 3 cm) are assigned 22 MELD exception points. Another 3 points are added for every additional 3-month waiting increment, reflecting a corresponding 10% increase in pretransplantation mortality risk.[45]

Bridging Therapy for Transplantation Candidates

"Dropout" due to HCC progression while waiting on the transplantation list is a significant problem. At 24 months, which can be a typical waiting time in some areas, the rate exceeds 40%.[48] Clinicians may resort to locally ablative strategies like radiofrequency ablation, percutaneous ethanol injection, TACE, or radioembolization and even surgery as temporizing measures to control or downstage the tumor prior to transplantation.[47] However, there are no randomized controlled data showing a survival benefit from these approaches.

■ Radiofrequency ablation (RFA) as a bridging strategy can decrease dropout rates[48] and has also produced favorable survival outcomes; in one series, the 3-year survival rate was 75%.[49]

■ The benefit of TACE as bridging therapy is controversial.[48] A recent meta-analysis reported that although pretransplantation TACE seems to be safe, it does not decrease dropout rates, increase eligibility for OLT, or improve overall survival.[50] TACE may be beneficial for treating larger, more advanced disease than RFA, but careful patient selection is required.

• The HeiLivCa trial is a phase III double-blinded, placebo-controlled study of carboplatin-based TACE with or without sorafenib as bridging therapy for patients awaiting transplantation.[51]

■ Patients whose disease previously exceeded the Milan and/or UCSF criteria may be downstaged sufficiently with transcatheter arterial radioembolization with ^{90}Y-radiolabeled microspheres to permit transplantation.[52–54]

- ^{90}Y-labeled microspheres are now being evaluated with or without sorafenib in a phase I study of transplantation-eligible patients (ClinicalTrials.gov, NCT00846131).

- Although the decision to proceed with bridging therapy depends on multiple factors, the waiting time for organ availability may influence the type of therapy and which patients should be treated.
  - One study suggested that patients whose estimated waiting time is between 4 and 9 months are most likely to benefit from TACE.[55]
  - Bridging surgery was determined to be cost effective and was associated with a 4.8- to 6.1-month survival advantage in transplantation candidates with an estimated waiting time of ≥ 1 year. Conversely, percutaneous ethanol injection was cost effective for all waiting times, but only increased life expectancy among those waiting for < 1 year.[56]

- Patients who exceed the Milan criteria can undergo bridging therapy followed by a 3- to 6-month observation period in order to downstage their disease and assess disease biology in vivo. Patients who respond well to these therapies or who progress despite them, may be spared an unnecessary surgery.[57]

- Some investigators have chosen to closely follow initially resected patients, reserving transplantation for salvage therapy at the time of relapse. Reports from different centers have been conflicting with respect to the efficacy and safety of this strategy.[58,59]

Living Donor Transplantation

- The shortage of organ donors is a major limiting factor affecting the availability of liver transplantation as a treatment option for HCC. In an attempt to address this issue, investigators have turned to living donor liver transplantation as an alternative.

- Data on living donor liver transplantation (LDLT) are mainly limited to retrospective cohort series, primarily in Asia. Results have been mixed, with different series reporting similar,[60] superior,[61] or inferior[62] outcomes for living compared to deceased donor liver transplantation (DDLT).

- Advantages of LDLT include shorter waiting periods, lower dropout rates, and shorter cold ischemic time, which would theoretically translate into improved outcomes.[63] Disadvantages include morbidity and mortality risks to both the donors and recipients.
  - The median morbidity rate for living donors is 16% and is mainly due to infectious and biliary complications.[64] The median mortality rate is 0.1–0.3%.[65]
  - In one series, the 3-year recurrence rates were significantly higher among LDLT versus DDLT recipients.[62] Although more patients undergoing LDLT exceeded the Milan criteria than in the DDLT group, the difference was not significant. A possible explanation is that LDLT patients had a more aggressive disease biology that would have manifested itself with a longer period of observation beforehand. Differences in surgical technique between transplantation of live versus cadaveric livers, as well as upregulation of proangiogenic and growth factors during surgery, may have also contributed to earlier recurrences.[63,66]
- There are no prospective data on the benefits of LDLT compared to DDLT. As with any intervention, risks and benefits must be considered, including those pertaining to the donor. LDLT should be performed at high-volume centers.

Comparing Outcomes for Transplantation and Partial Hepatectomy

- There are no randomized studies that have directly compared outcomes between transplanted and resected patients. However, retrospective data have indicated that OLT is the superior option for patients with cirrhosis and early HCC with respect to recurrence-free, disease-specific, and 5-year survival.[67,68] Nevertheless, these considerable benefits are counterbalanced by limited accessibility to resources and expertise, eligibility criteria struggling to balance safety and cost-effectiveness without being overly restrictive, and the need for immunosuppressive therapy with its implicit risks.

■ Nonsurgical Locally Ablative Therapies

Curative Strategies

▦ Medically unresectable patients with early-stage HCC are still potentially curable with locoregional ablative therapies.

Radiofrequency Ablation (RFA)

▦ Percutaneous or laparoscopically placed electrodes are inserted into tumors, causing coagulation necrosis by thermal energy conduction.

▦ Patients with Child-Pugh A or B cirrhosis with liver-confined disease are candidates.

▦ Success rates depend on size, location, and tumor multiplicity.

  • The best results are seen for lesions < 3.5 cm in diameter; ideally, the ablation field should be larger than the tumor.[69]

  • RFA is less effective for perivascular lesions since adjacent blood flow causes a "heat sink" effect resulting in rapid heat dissipation.[70]

  • In centers of expertise, patients with as many as five to six lesions measuring up to 7–8 cm in diameter have been successfully treated.[69]

▦ Adding liposomal doxorubicin to RFA may increase the volume of necrosis, allowing for the treatment of larger tumors, but this is still investigational.[71]

▦ Small studies in appropriately selected patients have demonstrated survival outcomes comparable to those achieved with surgery,[72,73] but these need to be confirmed in larger, randomized studies with long-term follow-up.

▦ Adverse events include a postembolization syndrome (right upper quadrant pain, fever, malaise, transaminitis) that usually resolves spontaneously within a week. In one series, liver abscesses were the predominant adverse event, followed by pleural effusion, skin burn, hypoxemia, pneumothorax, subcapsular hematoma, acute renal failure, hemoperitoneum, and needle tract seeding. The authors of this series also cautioned against the use of RFA in patients with portal vein thrombosis.[12]

Percutaneous Ethanol Injection (PEI)

▪ The injection of 95% ethanol into tumors causes both ischemic and cytotoxic necrosis. It was favored in the past as an inexpensive, simple, and effective procedure.[74]

▪ PEI is a reasonable and cost-effective option for patients with small (< 15–30 mm), well-differentiated tumors.[75,76] Larger lesions treated with PEI are associated with a higher risk of recurrence and are best treated surgically since the likelihood of long-term survival is also greater.[76]

▪ Randomized controlled data and meta-analyses have reported the superiority of RFA over PEI with respect to local disease control[77] and overall survival.[78] Complications, including hemothorax, hemoperitoneum, liver infarction, and abscess, are higher with RFA but are thought to be operator dependent.[78] Thus, for the most part, PEI has been supplanted by RFA.

Palliative Strategies

▪ Patients with intermediate-stage disease that is confined to the liver but unresectable can still achieve durable disease control and prolongation of survival with transarterial therapies.

Transcatheter Arterial Chemoembolization (TACE)

▪ The rationale for TACE and related techniques is based on the dependence of liver tumors on the hepatic artery for their blood supply, whereas normal liver parenchyma is primarily perfused by the portal vein. As such, chemotherapy can be selectively delivered to tumor tissue without damaging normal liver.

▪ Intra-arterial embolization of the hepatic artery causes hypoxia, with a compensatory increase in the expression of proangiogenic factors, tumor microvessel density, and antiapoptotic factors such as Bcl-2.[79–81] Chemotherapy is added in order to counteract these effects.[82] Tumor death thus occurs by cytotoxicity and ischemia.

▪ TACE is a palliative procedure for patients with larger and/or more advanced disease not amenable to RFA. Survival outcomes are predicted by the pretreatment

Child-Pugh score, > 50% liver involvement by tumor, and the presence of portal vein thrombosis.[83]

- The presence of portal vein thrombosis is often considered to be a contraindication for any intra-arterial embolic therapy. Embolization of the hepatic artery in the presence of a thrombosed portal vein can induce acute hepatic failure as a result of necrosis.[84,85]
  - Although the absence of vascular involvement is preferable, TACE can still be performed safely on selected patients with portal vein thrombosis but otherwise adequate hepatic reserve.[86]
- Chemotherapy drugs used in TACE should have a high hepatic extraction rate in order to minimize systemic exposure. Doxorubicin is the most commonly used drug but has been studied in combination with cisplatin and mitomycin.[87] No particular drug or combination has been shown to be better than the others.[88]
- Lipiodol, a poppy seed oil derivative, is a commonly used embolic substance that occludes the hepatic artery, thereby prolonging the intrahepatic concentration and duration of exposure to chemotherapy. Other embolic substances are gelatin-based or polyvinyl alcohol particles.[89]
- Two randomized controlled trials of patients with unresectable HCC, but preserved liver function, have shown a clear survival advantage with TACE over best supportive care.[90,91] These results were supported by a subsequent meta-analysis.[92] The completeness of response to TACE has been shown to correlate with survival in transplanted patients.[93]
- However, other meta-analyses have not shown any survival benefit to TACE compared to bland (i.e., without chemotherapy) transarterial embolization.[88,94] This might be due to the toxicity associated with TACE.[94]
- In addition to being a palliative measure, TACE has found a role at other points along the therapeutic spectrum for HCC, including as primary therapy for large, surgically and/or medically unresectable disease and also as bridge to liver transplantation (see above).

- Preoperative TACE has been evaluated, but this practice is discouraged. Several studies have indicated an association with poorer survival, partly because it delays surgery and complicates the management of future recurrences.[95,96]
- The toxicities associated with TACE are similar to those described for RFA, with postembolization syndrome being the most frequent side effect. Post-TACE hepatic decompensation is a rare but real concern, again underscoring the need for careful patient selection because the risk is associated with greater underlying hepatic dysfunction.[97]

Doxorubicin-Eluting Bead (DEB)-TACE

- DEB-TACE offers the advantages of controlled drug release and reduced systemic toxicity and is an alternative to conventional TACE.[98]
- In a randomized, international, multicenter phase II study directly comparing the two techniques, nonsignificant trends toward better response and disease control rates were observed in the DEB-TACE cohort. Among those with more unfavorable characteristics (Child-Pugh B cirrhosis, recurrent or bilobar disease, Eastern Cooperative Oncology Group [ECOG] performance status = 1), the difference was significant.[99]
  - DEB-TACE also had a better toxicity profile than conventional TACE. Systemic side effects, including alopecia, skin discoloration, mucositis, and myelosuppression, were significantly lower and less severe with DEB-TACE, as were hepatotoxicity and cardiotoxicity. The incidence of postembolization syndrome was similar.[99]
- A retrospective review reported a significant survival advantage with DEB-TACE over conventional TACE, but only in patients with Child-Pugh A/B cirrhosis, a Cancer of the Liver Italian Program (CLIP) score ≤ 3, and Okuda stage I disease. Survival was similar between patients with and without portal vein thrombosis within the DEB-TACE group, although no comparisons were made with conventional TACE.[100]

- A prospective randomized trial also reported significant improvements in response rates, time to progression, and decreased recurrences with DEB-TACE compared with bland transarterial embolization. One-year survival was 85% for both groups (see below).[82]
- An additional benefit of DEB-TACE is that drug loading can be done accurately and does not affect handling and delivery of the beads. Treatment preparation can therefore be done in a standardized manner.[101]

Bland Transarterial Embolization (TAE)

- It is often difficult to separate the relative contributions of cytotoxicity and ischemia to tumor death caused by TACE, although some investigators believe that ischemia is the predominant mechanism. In an attempt to eliminate the systemic toxicities associated with TACE, bland embolization (i.e., without chemotherapy) or TAE has been explored.
  - In a single-institution review of patients with unresectable HCC treated with TAE, median survival was 21 months with 1-, 2-, and 3-year survival rates of 66%, 46%, and 33%, respectively. When patients with extrahepatic metastases or portal vein involvement were excluded, the median survival rose to 40 months with 1-, 2-, and 3-year survival rates of 84%, 66%, and 51%, respectively.[102]
- The relative efficacy of TAE compared to TACE has not been adequately addressed prospectively, and data are conflicting. Although some studies suggest that the two approaches have comparable efficacy,[88,94] others report that TACE is superior to TAE.[82] The single randomized, prospective trial comparing both techniques to supportive care was terminated early when a significant survival benefit emerged favoring TACE over the control group. Although no significant differences in survival were seen between the TACE and TAE groups, a formal analysis was not performed.[91]
  - Compared to TACE, TAE has been associated with lower rates of periprocedural morbidity and mortality.[94]

- Data comparing TAE to best supportive care demonstrate superior tumor responses but no survival benefit.[92,103] However, these studies may have been inadequately powered to detect a difference.
- An important consideration with bland embolization is particle size; smaller particles can reach terminal vessels, which is necessary to achieve more selective as well as more complete tumor necrosis.[102] Small spherical or nonspherical polyvinyl alcohol particles cause permanent vessel occlusion and are currently preferred over the gelatin-based particles, which only cause temporary occlusion.[88]

Radiotherapy and Radioembolization

- The exquisite radiosensitivity of the liver parenchyma has limited the use of external-beam radiotherapy in the treatment of HCC, although high, durable response rates can be achieved.[104] Technical refinements in the delivery of external-beam radiotherapy and the development of radioembolization have maintained this treatment modality as a viable and valuable adjunct to surgery and other locoregional therapies.
- Transcatheter arterial radioembolization (TARE) is analogous to TACE. Instead of chemotherapy, ^{90}Y-embedded glass or resin microspheres are used to selectively irradiate tumor tissue while sparing the normal liver parenchyma.
- In a prospective cohort study, objective response rates were 40–60% and survival was up to 17.2 months in patients with Child-Pugh A cirrhosis.[105] Patients with more advanced cirrhosis, lymph node or extrahepatic disease, and portal vein thrombosis have poorer outcomes with TARE.[105,106] Patient selection criteria, as well as the clinical applications of TARE, thus mirror those of TACE.
- Unlike TACE, TARE causes less ischemic necrosis because the microspheres do not completely occlude the hepatic artery. Therefore, there is less of a risk for ischemic hepatic failure because some perfusion is maintained. Recent prospective and retrospective studies have

reported the efficacy and acceptable safety of TARE in patients with portal vein thrombosis.[85,105,107]

- Advantages of TARE over TACE include being able to perform TARE in the outpatient setting and fewer treatments to achieve the same effect.[89] However, randomized controlled studies with long-term follow-up comparing TARE to TACE and other therapies are lacking.

- Intensity-modulated, stereotactic body[108] and proton beam radiotherapy[109,110] techniques have been developed to improve the therapeutic index of external-beam radiotherapy.[112] Conformal radiotherapy has also been investigated as a bridging therapy to liver transplantation and appears to be both safe and effective.[112] The role of these techniques in the management of HCC continues to be evaluated.

- The growing array of locoregional therapies offers the possibility of durable disease control, prolongation of survival, and depending on the extent of disease, cure for patients who are not surgical candidates. In general, those who benefit the most from these therapies have a good performance status, preserved liver function, and liver-confined disease. Selected patients with portal vein thrombosis may also be able to undergo intra-arterial embolic therapy or radiotherapy. Ultimately, the choice of therapy depends on the clinical picture, an informed patient decision, and the local expertise.

■ Systemic Therapy

- Patients with extensive locally advanced and/or widespread metastatic disease are treated systemically with palliative intent; the goals being symptom and disease control, prolongation of survival, and improvement of quality of life. Targeted therapies such as sorafenib have, in recent years, changed the landscape for the management of advanced HCC and will be the focus of this section. Historical treatments including chemotherapy, immunotherapy, and hormonal therapy have been studied extensively but have failed to show a meaningful improvement in survival.

Chemotherapy

▣ HCC is a fairly chemotherapy-resistant tumor due to the overexpression of drug resistance genes including multidrug resistance (*MDR1*) gene and P-glycoprotein.[113] Furthermore, the underlying hepatic dysfunction present in most patients limits the therapeutic index of chemotherapy.

▣ No single agent or combination of chemotherapy has been approved by the Food and Drug Administration (FDA) for the treatment of HCC.

▣ Initial enthusiasm for doxorubicin based on a single study demonstrating a response rate of 79%[114] has been tempered by subsequent data showing a much smaller margin of benefit. Typical response rates average around 15–20%, with a median survival of only 4 months.[115] Systematic reviews have shown no evidence of a survival benefit to justify the toxicities.[116] Although combination therapy, often with cisplatin, does produce higher response rates, the benefits are short-lived and do not support its routine use over single-agent therapy.[117]

▣ Other agents including gemcitabine,[118] fluoropyrimidines,[119,120] and irinotecan[121] have shown response or disease control rates of approximately 25%, but these have not been consistently reproduced or found to be durable.

▣ Combination regimens with platinum agents like cisplatin and oxaliplatin appear to confer added activity, but do not improve survival.[122,123]

  • Gemcitabine and oxaliplatin produced a disease control rate of 76% including partial responses in 18% of patients. Median progression-free and overall survival times were 6.3 and 11.5 months, respectively. Patients with nonalcoholic cirrhosis benefitted more compared to those with alcoholic cirrhosis.[124]

Chemoimmunotherapy with Interferon-Alfa (IFN-α)

▣ In a single study of 50 patients with unresectable or metastatic HCC, the PIAF regimen (cisplatin, IFN-α, doxorubicin, and 5-fluorouracil) produced pathologic complete responses and induced remissions in approximately 10% and

20% of patients, respectively. However, grade ≥ 3 hematologic toxicities were significant, and two patients died of neutropenic sepsis. Median overall survival was 8.9 months.[125]

- A randomized phase III trial of PIAF versus doxorubicin showed a better objective response rate with PIAF, but at the expense of more toxicity without any survival benefit.[126]
- As previously mentioned, PIAF has shown activity in the neoadjuvant setting.[27]
- Chemoimmunotherapy cannot be considered a standard approach for advanced HCC in view of its toxicity, limited efficacy, and unremarkable impact on survival when compared to the newer targeted agents that are currently available (see Targeted Therapy). The results with neoadjuvant PIAF appear promising, but require further investigation and judicious patient selection.

Hormonal Therapy

- The discovery of constitutively active variant estrogen receptors[127] suggested a potential therapeutic role for tamoxifen in HCC. However, systematic reviews have consistently shown no evidence of benefit.[128]
- Although some HCCs express somatostatin receptors,[129] randomized controlled data have not shown any survival advantage with octreotide in advanced HCC.[130]

Targeted Therapy

Sorafenib

- Sorafenib is an orally administrated small-molecule tyrosine kinase inhibitor of the Raf/MEK/Erk pathway, as well as the intracellular domains of vascular endothelial growth factor receptor (VEGFR), platelet-derived growth factor receptor (PDGFR), c-kit, FLT3, and Ret.[131]
- The activity of sorafenib in advanced HCC was initially evaluated in a phase II study that documented significant improvements in median time to progression and overall survival despite a very modest objective response rate of 8%.[132]
- The randomized, placebo-controlled phase III Sorafenib HCC Assessment Randomized Protocol (SHARP) trial confirmed the significant benefits of sorafenib with

respect to overall survival and time to radiographic progression. The toxicity profile of sorafenib was acceptable with grade 3 hypertension, abdominal pain, diarrhea, and hand-foot syndrome occurring in 2–8% of patients. [133]

- A subsequent phase III Asian study reported similar findings, albeit to a smaller degree than in the SHARP trial. [134] Patients in the Asian trial had a poorer performance status and more advanced disease at enrollment, which might partly explain this observation. In addition, post hoc subgroup analyses suggest that hepatitis B virus (HBV) infection, which is more prevalent in Asian countries, is associated with a lesser response to sorafenib than in patients with hepatitis C virus (HCV). [135,136] The outcomes of patients with HBV on the SHARP trial have not been presented.

Sorafenib and Liver Dysfunction

- Clinical experience regarding the safety of sorafenib in patients with more advanced hepatic dysfunction is limited. Retrospective analyses of patients with Child-Pugh B or C cirrhosis report poorer responses and a high risk of hepatic decompensation. [137–139] Initial dose reductions are indicated depending on the degree of hyperbilirubinemia and hypoalbuminemia. [140]
  - Patients with a total bilirubin ≤ 1.5× the upper limit of normal (ULN), an elevated aspartate transaminase (AST), and a creatinine clearance (CrCl) of 40–59 mL/min can still receive the full dose of sorafenib at 400 mg orally (PO) twice a day (BID).
  - Those with a total bilirubin of 1.5–3× ULN, any AST, or CrCl of 20–39 mL/min should receive 200 mg PO BID.
  - Patients with a serum albumin < 2.5 mg/dL or who are on dialysis can receive 200 mg PO once a day.
  - Patients with bilirubin of 3–10× ULN are unlikely to tolerate sorafenib at 200 mg PO every third day and probably should not be treated.

Sorafenib and Doxorubicin

- The potential to improve upon the results seen with sorafenib monotherapy was suggested in a randomized phase II trial of doxorubicin ± sorafenib.[141] Response rates were low at 2–4%, but overall survival was doubled with combination therapy (13.7 vs. 6.5 months, P = .02). The median time to progression and progression-free survival were also significantly increased with combination therapy. The phase III Cancer and Leukemia Group B (CALGB) 80802 trial evaluating sorafenib ± doxorubicin is currently under way and is open at multiple centers across North America (ClinicalTrials.gov, NCT01015833).

Sorafenib & TACE

- Sorafenib has also been combined with TACE with the hope of delaying tumor recurrence or progression and to prevent liver damage incurred by repeated TACE treatments. A phase III trial randomizing patients post-TACE to sorafenib or placebo did not show an improvement in time to progression with the combination.[144] It has been speculated that sorafenib was given too late to coincide with the transient upregulation of proangiogenic factors post-TACE. Furthermore, the number of TACE treatments and duration of sorafenib were felt to be suboptimal.[143]
  - The combination of embolization and sorafenib given on a continuous schedule has proven its safety but is awaiting the results of several randomized trials (e.g., ECOG 2108 and SPACE) to study its efficacy.[145]

Anti–Epidermal Growth Factor Receptor (EGFR) Agents

- Agents targeting various components of the EGFR pathway including the extracellular domain of the receptor (cetuximab, lapatinib) and the tyrosine kinase domain (lapatinib, erlotinib) have shown only modest antitumor activity.[144,146–148]
- The insulin/insulin-like growth factor axis, hepatocyte growth factor, and the c-MET receptor are other members of the EGFR family. Inhibition of these pathways has shown antitumor activity in vitro[149,150] and is also currently being investigated in multiple phase I and II clinical trials (ClinicalTrials.gov, NCT00639509, NCT00906373, NCT01101906).[151]

Antiangiogenic Agents

- Bevacizumab, a monoclonal antibody against the vascular endothelial growth factor (VEGF), has been the most actively studied antiangiogenic agent. It has shown single-agent activity in phase II trials, albeit with significant adverse events including one death due to hemorrhaging from esophageal varices.[152,153]
    - Bevacizumab combined with gemcitabine and oxaliplatin,[154] capecitabine alone,[155] or capecitabine and oxaliplatin[156] has also shown activity, but at the expense of increased toxicity.
    - The combination of bevacizumab and erlotinib appears promising. A quarter of patients had partial responses, 37% had stable disease, progression-free survival at 16 weeks was 62.5%, and the median overall survival time was 15.6 months.[157] Bevacizumab and erlotinib are now being evaluated against sorafenib in a randomized phase II trial (ClinicalTrials.gov, NCT00881751).
    - An important consideration in patients with cirrhosis and portal hypertension being treated with bevacizumab is the risk of fatal variceal hemorrhaging. Patients must therefore undergo endoscopy and be treated for varices before beginning bevacizumab.[152,158]
- Sunitinib, a multitargeted tyrosine kinase inhibitor similar to sorafenib, has shown only modest activity in phase II studies. Objective response rates have been < 3%, and reported median progression-free and overall survival times are approximately 4 and 10 months, respectively.[159,160] Toxicities including encephalopathy, myelosuppression, and bleeding events were concerning. A phase III trial comparing sorafenib with sunitinib was terminated early due to excess toxicity and failure of sunitinib to demonstrate superiority or noninferiority with respect to overall survival.[161]
- Other antiangiogenic agents targeting VEGF as well as fibroblast growth factor (FGF) and platelet-derived growth factor (PDGF) such as ABT869[162] and brivanib[163] have shown single-agent activity in phase II trials and are currently being evaluated in phase III trials against sorafenib (ClinicalTrials.gov, NCT00858871, NCT0100959).

Downstream Signaling Pathways

- The two major pathways are the Ras/Raf/Mek/Erk and PI3K/Akt/mTOR signaling cascades.
- Farnesyltransferase is required to activate Ras.[164] 3-hydroxy-3-methylglutaryl-coenzyme A reductase inhibitors like statins suppress farnesyltransferase[165] and are currently being evaluated in clinical trials (ClinicalTrials.gov, NCT01075555), as are direct farnesyltransferase inhibitors (ClinicalTrials.gov, NCT00020774).
- Mammalian target of rapamycin (mTOR) inhibitors like sirolimus have been shown to reduce the risk of recurrences in patients who have undergone liver transplantation for HCC.[166–169] This class of agents is now being prospectively evaluated in multiple phase I, II, and III trials.

■ Special Considerations in Assessing Treatment Responses in HCC

- Response Evaluation Criteria in Solid Tumors (RECIST) guidelines quantify changes in unidimensional tumor measurements to determine responses to therapy. These criteria do not adequately capture the activity of targeted agents, many of which are cytostatic in contrast to cytotoxic chemotherapy. In this case, disease stabilization could represent a "response." This may explain why a survival benefit was still seen with sorafenib in the SHARP trial despite the relative absence of objective responses (2% partial responses, 0% complete responses).[133]
- The extent of tumor viability is being increasingly recognized as a more important and reliable indicator of response than tumor shrinkage. Patients who responded to sorafenib demonstrated a significant increase in tumor necrosis relative to tumor volume from baseline on CT scans.[170] In some cases, tumor dimension actually increased due to reactive inflammation and edema.[132] Changes in the ratio of tumor necrosis to tumor volume as biomarkers of response to sorafenib require prospective validation.
- The American Association for the Study of Liver Disease (AASLD) has developed modified RECIST criteria that

include an assessment of tumor tissue viability based on the amount of intratumoral contrast uptake during the arterial phase of dynamic imaging studies.[171] A limitation of these criteria is that changes in intratumoral enhancement may result from the effects of antiangiogenic therapies on tumor vasculature without reflecting actual antitumor activity.[171] Prospective validation, possibly with biopsy confirmation, is required before modified RECIST criteria can be fully adopted in clinical practice.

◾ New response evaluation criteria have also been developed for locoregional ablative therapies in HCC. In 2000, the European Association for the Study of Liver (EASL) recommended that the reduction in viable tumor volume be used to determine responses.[172] Advantages of the EASL criteria include early response detection (within 1.6 months), as well as predictive potential with respect to survival.[173,174] As with other newer response criteria, prospective validation is required.

◾ Advances in dynamic imaging techniques such as diffusion-weighted MRI, blood oxygen level–dependent (BOLD) MRI, image subtraction, and functional MRI (see Chapter 3) can also help to optimize response evaluation to locoregional ablative therapies.

◼ Antiviral Therapy in the Management of HCC

HBV Carriers

◾ Reactivation of HBV in chronic carriers is a major concern that has been associated with deleterious outcomes in patients with HCC or non-HCC tumors who are undergoing anticancer therapy.[175–178]

◾ In a prospective study of 102 patients with advanced HCC receiving PIAF or doxorubicin, 58% developed hepatitis, of which 37% of cases were due to HBV reactivation. Hepatitis was more severe in patients with reactivation compared to those without. The mortality rate from reactivated HBV was 30%, although median survival was not significantly different between patients with and without reactivation.[177]

- A high pretreatment HBV viral load has been associated with more severe hepatitis on therapy and appears to be an independent risk factor for poor survival.[179]
- HBV reactivation from chemotherapy-induced immunosuppression is preventable with antiviral therapy, thus supporting a role for screening.[178] A recent prospective study at Memorial Sloan-Kettering Cancer Center (MSKCC) found that only 50% of patients seropositive for HBsAg or HBcAb came from endemic areas.[180] Therefore, all patients seen at MSKCC, regardless of race or country of origin, are now routinely screened and treated where indicated before beginning anticancer therapy. However, this is not accepted as standard practice at all institutions.

HCV Carriers

- Although HCV reactivation has been well documented in patients undergoing therapy for hematologic malignancies, its occurrence in patients being treated for solid malignancies is rare.[181–183]
- Potential mechanisms leading to reactivation can occur due to immunosuppression or immune reconstitution following the end of chemotherapy.[181,182]

■ Treatment of Mixed Cholangiocarcinoma-Hepatocellular Carcinoma (CC-HCC)

- Aggressive surgical resection provides the best possibility of cure and long-term survival.[185,186] In one series, the median and 5-year survival rates were 32 months and 24%, respectively. In contrast, the median survival for patients with unresectable CC-HCC was 18 months.[185]
- Liver transplantation has also been reported as another potentially curative measure for CC-HCC, although experience is extremely limited.[186,187] Survival up to 25 to 35 months has been reported.[187]
- There is no standard of care for the management of recurrent or advanced disease. Systemic chemotherapy may be considered as well as locoregional therapies such as cryoablation or RFA. Intra-arterial embolic therapies are less

likely to be effective in CC-HCC tumors because they are less vascular and more fibrotic than pure HCCs.[185,188]

■ References

1. Llovet JM, Bru C, Bruix J. Prognosis of hepatocellular carcinoma: the BCLC staging classification. *Semin Liver Dis* 1999;19:329–338.

2. Vauthey J-N, Dixon E, Abdalla EK, et al. Pretreatment assessment of hepatocellular carcinoma: expert consensus statement. *HPB* 2010;12:289–299.

3. Yamanaka N, Okamoto E, Toyosaka A, et al. Prognostic factors after hepatectomy for hepatocellular carcinomas. A univariate and multivariate analysis. *Cancer* 1990;65:1104–1110.

4. Vauthey N, Klimstra D, Franceschi D, et al. Factors affecting outcome after hepatic resection for hepatocellular carcinoma. *Am J Surg* 1995;169:28–34.

5. Takayama T, Makuuchi M, Hirohashi S, et al. Early hepatocellular carcinoma as an entity with a high rate of surgical cure. *Hepatology* 1998;28:1241–1246.

6. Belghiti J, Panis Y, Farges O, et al. Intrahepatic recurrence after resection of hepatocellular carcinoma complicating cirrhosis. *Ann Surg* 1991;214:114–117.

7. Molmenti EP, Klintmalm GB. Liver transplantation in association with hepatocellular carcinoma: an update of the International Tumor Registry. *Liver Transpl* 2002;8:736–748.

8. Bruix J, Castells A, Bosch J, et al. Surgical resection of hepatocellular carcinoma in cirrhotic patients: prognostic value of preoperative portal pressure. *Gastroenterology* 1996;111:1018–1022.

9. Abrams P, Walsh JW. Current approach to hepatocellular carcinoma. *Surg Clin North Am* 2010;90:803–816.

10. Singal AK, Ahmad M, Soloway RD. Duplex Doppler ultrasound examination of the portal venous system: an emerging novel technique for the estimation of portal vein pressure. *Dig Dis Sci* 2010;55:1230–1240.

11. Vauthey JN, Chaoui A, Do KA, et al. Standardized measurement of the future liver remnant prior to extended liver resection: methodology and clinical associations. *Surgery* 2000;127:512–519.

12. de Baere T, Roche A, Elias D, et al. Preoperative portal vein embolization for extension of hepatectomy indications. *Hepatology* 1996;24:1386–1391.

13. Urata K, Kawasaki S, Matsunami H, et al. Calculation of child and adult standard liver volume for liver transplantation. *Hepatology* 1995;21:1317–1321.

14. Abulkhir A, Limongelli P, Healey AJ, et al. Preoperative portal vein embolization for major liver resection: a meta-analysis. *Ann Surg* 2008;247:49–57.

15. Fan J, Tang ZY, Yu YQ, et al. Improved survival with resection after transcatheter arterial chemoembolization (TACE) for unresectable hepatocellular carcinoma. *Dig Surg* 1998;15: 674–678.

16. Adachi E, Matsumata T, Nishizaki, et al. Effects of preoperative transcatheter hepatic arterial chemoembolization for hepatocellular carcinoma. The relationship between postoperative course and tumor necrosis. *Cancer* 1993;72: 3593–3598.

17. Choi GH, Kim DH, Kang CM, et al. Is preoperative transarterial chemoembolization needed for a resectable hepatocellular carcinoma? *World J Surg* 2007;32:2370–2377.

18. Lee KT, Lu YW, Wang SN, et al. The effect of preoperative transarterial chemoembolization of resectable hepatocellular carcinoma on clinical and economic outcomes. *J Surg Oncol* 2009;99:343–350.

19. Sasaki A, Iwashita Y, Shibata K, et al. Preoperative transcatheter arterial chemoembolization reduces long-term survival rate after hepatic resection for resectable hepatocellular carcinoma. *EJSO* 2006;32:773–779.

20. Luo YQ, Wang Y, Chen H, et al. Influence of preoperative transcatheter arterial chemoembolization on liver resection in patients with resectable hepatocellular carcinoma. *Hepatobiliary Pancreat Dis Int* 2002;1:523–526.

21. Uchida M, Kohno H, Kubota H, et al. Role of preoperative transcatheter arterial oily chemoembolization for resectable hepatocellular carcinoma. *World J Surg* 1996;20:326–331.

22. Ogata S, Belghiti J, Farges O, et al. Sequential arterial and portal vein embolizations before right hepatectomy in patients with cirrhosis and hepatocellular carcinoma. *Br J Surg* 2006;93:1091–1098.

23. Aoki T, Imamura H, Hasegawa K, et al. Sequential preoperative arterial and portal venous embolizations in patients with hepatocellular carcinoma. *Arch Surg* 2004;139:766–774.

24. Sitzmann JV, Abrams R. Improved survival for hepatocellular cancer with combination surgery and multimodality treatment. *Ann Surg* 1993;217:149–154.

25. Lau WY, Ho S, Leung TW, et al. Selective internal radiation therapy for nonresectable hepatocellular carcinoma with intraarterial infusion of 90 yttrium microspheres. *Int J Radiat Oncol Biol Phys* 1998;40:583–592.

26. Raoul JL, Messner M, Boucher E, et al. Preoperative treatment of hepatocellular carcinoma with intra-arterial injection of 131I-labelled lipiodol. *Br J Surg* 2003;90:1379–1383.

27. Lau WY, Leung TW, Lai BS, et al. Preoperative systemic chemoimmunotherapy and sequential resection for unresectable hepatocellular carcinoma. *Ann Surg* 2001;233:236–241.

28. Lau WY, Ho SK, Yu SC, et al. Salvage surgery following downstaging of unresectable hepatocellular carcinoma. *Ann Surg* 2004;240:299–305.

29. Tang ZY, Yu YQ, Zhou XD, et al. Cytoreduction and sequential resection for surgically verified unresectable hepatocellular carcinoma: evaluation with analysis of 72 patients. *World J Surg* 1995;19:784–789.

30. Nonami T, Isshiki K, Katoh H, et al. The potential role of postoperative hepatic artery chemotherapy in patients with high-risk hepatomas. *Ann Surg* 1991;213:222–226.

31. Ono T, Yamanoi A, Nazmy El-Assal O, et al. Adjuvant chemotherapy after resection of hepatocellular carcinoma causes deterioration of long-term prognosis in cirrhotic patients: metaanalysis of three randomized controlled trials. *Cancer* 2001;91:2378–2385.

32. Xia Y, Ziu Y, Li J, et al. Adjuvant therapy with capecitabine postpones recurrence of hepatocellular carcinoma after curative resection: a randomized controlled trial. *Ann Surg Oncol* 2010;17:3137–3144.

33. Lau YW, Lai EC, Leung TW, et al. Adjuvant intra-arterial iodine-131-labeled lipiodol for resectable hepatocellular carcinoma: a prospective randomized trial-update on 5-year and 10-year survival. *Ann Surg* 2008;247:43–48.

34. Boucher E, Corbinais S, Rolland Y, et al. Adjuvant intra-arterial injection of iodine-131-labeled lipiodol after resection of hepatocellular carcinoma. *Hepatology* 2003;38:1237–1240.

35. Zhou GD, Richardson M, Fasili IS, et al. Role of retinoic acid in the modulation of benzo(a)pyrene-DNA adducts in human hepatoma cells: implications for cancer prevention. *Toxicol Appl Pharmacol* 2010;249:224–230.

36. Muto Y, Moriwaki H, Ninomiya M, et al. Prevention of second primary tumors by an acyclic retinoid, polyprenoic acid, in patients with hepatocellular carcinoma. *N Engl J Med* 1996;334:1561–1568.

37. Muto Y, Moriwaki H, Saito A, et al. Prevention of second primary tumors by an acyclic retinoid in patients with hepatocellular carcinoma. *N Engl J Med* 1999;340:1046–1047.

38. Okita K, Matsui O, Kumada H, et al. Effect of peretinoin on recurrence of hepatocellular carcinoma (HCC): results of a phase II/III randomized placebo-controlled trial [abstract]. *J Clin Oncol* 2010;28(suppls 15s):4024.

39. Mazzafero V, Regalia E, Doci R, et al. Liver transplantation for the treatment of small hepatocellular carcinomas in patients with cirrhosis. *N Engl J Med* 1996;334:693–699.

40. Mazzaferro V, Llovet JM, Miceli R, et al. Predicting survival after liver transplantation in patients with hepatocellular carcinoma beyond the Milan criteria: a retrospective, exploratory analysis. *Lancet Oncol* 2009;10:35–43.

41. Yao FL, Ferrell L, Bass NM, et al. Liver transplantation for hepatocellular carcinoma: expansion of the tumor size limits does not adversely impact survival. *Hepatology* 2001;33: 1394–1403.

42. Decaens T, Roudot-Thoraval F, Hadni-Bresson S, et al. Impact of UCSF criteria according to pre- and post-OLT tumor features: analysis of 479 patients listed for HCC with a short waiting time. *Liver Transpl* 2006;12:1761–1769.

43. Mazzaferro V. Results of liver transplantation: with or without Milan criteria? *Liver Transpl* 2007;13(Suppl 2):S44–S47.

44. Kamath PS, Wiesner RH, Malinchoc M, et al. A model to predict survival in patients with end-stage liver disease. *Hepatology* 2001;33:464–470.

45. Freeman RB, Wiesner RH, Edwards E, et al. Results of the first year of the new liver allocation plan. *Liver Transpl* 2004; 10:7–15.

46. Yao FY, Bass NM, Nikolai B, et al. Liver transplantation for hepatocellular carcinoma: analysis of survival according to the intention-to-treat principle and dropout from the waiting list. *Liver Transpl* 2002;10:873–883.

47. Yao FY, Hirose R, LaBerge JM, et al. A prospective study on downstaging of hepatocellular carcinoma prior to liver transplantation. *Liver Transpl* 2005;11:1505–1514.

48. Lee FT. Treatment of hepatocellular carcinoma in cirrhosis: locoregional therapies for bridging to liver transplant. *Liver Transpl* 2007;13(Suppl 2):S24–S26.

49. Lu DS, Yu NC, Raman SS, et al. Percutaneous radiofrequency ablation of hepatocellular carcinoma as a bridge to liver transplantation. *Hepatology* 2005;41:1130–1137.

50. Lesurtel M, Mullhaupt B, Pestalozzi BC, et al. Transarterial chemoembolization as a bridge to liver transplantation for hepatocellular carcinoma: an evidence-based analysis. *Am J Transpl* 2006;6:2644.

51. Hoffman K, Glimm H, Radeleff B, et al. Prospective, randomized, double-blind, multi-center, phase III clinical study on transarterial chemoembolization (TACE) combined with sorafenib versus TACE plus placebo in patients with hepatocellular cancer before liver transplantation: HeiLivCa [ISRC TN24081794]. *BMC Cancer* 2008;26:349.

52. Ettorre GM, Santoro R, Puoti C, et al. Short-term follow-up of radioembolization with yttrium-90 microspheres before liver transplantation: new perspectives in advanced hepatocellular carcinoma. *Transplantation* 2010;90:930–931.

53. Kim DY, Kwon DS, Salem R, et al. Successful embolization of hepatocellular carcinoma with yttrium-90 glass microspheres prior to liver transplantation. *J Gastrointest Surg* 2006;10:413–416.

54. Khalaf H, Alsuhaibani H, Al-Sugair A, et al. Use of yttrium-90 microsphere radioembolization of hepatocellular carcinoma as downstaging and bridge before liver transplantation: a case report. *Transpl Proc* 2010;42:994–998.

55. Aloia TA, Adam R, Samuel D, et al. A decision analysis model identifies the interval of efficacy for transarterial chemoembolization (TACE) in cirrhotic patients with hepatocellular carcinoma awaiting liver transplantation. *J Gastrointest Surg* 2007;11:1328–1332.

56. Llovet JM, Mas X, Aponte JJ, et al. Cost effectiveness of adjuvant therapy for hepatocellular carcinoma during the waiting list for liver transplantation. *Gut* 2002;50:123–128.

57. Jarnagin W, Chapman WC, Curley S, et al. Surgical treatment of hepatocellular carcinoma: expert consensus statement. *HPB* 2010;12:302–310.

58. Belghiti J, Cortes A, Abdalla EK, et al. Resection prior to liver transplantation for hepatocellular carcinoma. *Ann Surg* 2003;238:885–892.

59. Cherqui D, Laurent A, Mocellin N, et al. Liver resection for transplantable hepatocellular carcinoma: long-term survival and role of secondary liver transplantation. *Ann Surg* 2009; 250:738–746.

60. Li C, Wen TF, Yan LN, et al. Outcome of hepatocellular carcinoma treated by liver transplantation: comparison of living donor and deceased donor transplantation. *Hepatobiliary Pancreat Dis Int* 2010;9:366–369.

61. Lo CM, Fan ST, Liu CL, et al. The role and limitation of living donor liver transplantation for hepatocellular carcinoma. *Liver Transpl* 2004;10:440–447.

62. Fisher RA, Kulik LM, Friese CE, et al. Hepatocellular carcinoma recurrence and death following living and deceased donor liver transplantation. *Am J Transplant* 2007;7: 1601–1608.

63. Kaido T, Uemoto S. Does living donation have advantages over deceased donation in liver transplantation? *J Gastroenterol Hepatol* 2010;25:1598–1603.

64. Middleton PF, Duffield M, Lynch SV, et al. Living donor transplantation-adult donor outcomes: a systematic review. *Liver Transpl* 2006;12:24–30.

65. Ringe B, Strong BW. The dilemma of living donor death: to report or not to report? *Transplantation* 2008;85:790–793.

66. Ninomiya M, Harada N, Shiotani S, et al. Hepatocyte growth factor and transforming growth factor beta1 contribute to

regeneration of small-for-size liver graft immediately after transplantation. *Transpl Int* 2003;16:814–819.

67. Bismuth H, Chiche L, Adam R, et al. Liver resection versus transplantation for hepatocellular carcinoma in cirrhotic patients. *Ann Surg* 1993;218:145–151.

68. Colella G, Botelli R, De Carlis L, et al. Hepatocellular carcinoma: comparison between liver transplantation, resective surgery, ethanol injection, and chemoembolization. *Transpl Int* 1998;11(Suppl 1):S193–S196.

69. Tanabe KK, Curley SA, Dodd GD, et al. Radiofrequency ablation: the experts weight in. *Cancer* 2004;100:641–650.

70. Huang J, Li T, Liu N, et al. Safety and reliability of hepatic radiofrequency ablation near the inferior vena cava: an experimental study. *Int J Hyperthermia* 2011;27:116–123.

71. Goldberg SN, Kamel IR, Kruskal JB, et al. Radiofrequency ablation of hepatic tumors: increased tumor destruction with adjuvant liposomal doxorubicin therapy. *AJR Am J Roentgenol* 2002;179:93–101.

72. Chen MS, Li JQ, Zheng Y, et al. A prospective randomized trial comparing percutaneous local ablative therapy and partial hepatectomy for small hepatocellular carcinoma. *Ann Surg* 2006;243:321–328.

73. Livraghi T, Meloni F, Di Stasi M, et al. Sustained complete response and complications rates after radiofrequency ablation of very early hepatocellular carcinoma in cirrhosis: is resection still the treatment of choice? *Hepatology* 2008;47:82–89.

74. Livraghi T, Bolondi L, Lazzaroni S, et al. Percutaneous ethanol injection in the treatment of hepatocellular carcinoma in cirrhosis. A study on 207 patients. *Cancer* 1992;69:925–929.

75. Hasegawa S, Yamasaki N, Hiwaki T, et al. Factors that predict intrahepatic recurrence of hepatocellular carcinoma in 81 patients initially treated by percutaneous ethanol injection. *Cancer* 1999;86:1682–1690.

76. Gournay J, Tchuenbou J, Richou C, et al. Percutaneous ethanol injection vs. resection in patients with small single hepatocellular carcinoma: a retrospective case-control study with cost analysis. *Aliment Pharmacol Ther* 2002;16:1529–1538.

77. Lencioni RA, Allgaier HP, Cioni D, et al. Small hepatocellular carcinoma in cirrhosis: randomized comparison of radio-frequency thermal ablation versus percutaneous ethanol injection. *Radiology* 2003;228:235–240.

78. Bouza C, Lopez-Cuadrado T, Alcazar R, et al. Meta-analysis of percutaneous radiofrequency ablation versus ethanol injection in hepatocellular carcinoma. *BMC Gastroenterol* 2009;9:31.

79. Virmani S, Rhee TK, Ryu RK, et al. Comparison of hypoxia-inducible factor-1alpha expression before and

after transcatheter arterial embolization in rabbit VX2 liver tumors. *J Vasc Interv Radiol* 2008;19:1483–1489.

80. Kobayashi N, Ishii M, Ueno Y, et al. Co-expression of Bcl-2 protein and vascular endothelial growth factor in hepatocellular carcinomas treated by chemoembolization. *Liver* 1999; 19:25–31.

81. Liao XF, Yi JL, Li XR, et al. Angiogenesis in rabbit hepatic tumor after transcatheter arterial embolization. *World J Gastroenterol* 2004;10:1885–1889.

82. Malagari K, Pomoni M, Kelekis A, et al. Prospective randomized comparison of chemoembolization with doxorubicin-eluting beads and bland embolization with BeadBlock for hepatocellular carcinoma. *Cardiovasc Intervent Radiol* 2010;33:541–551.

83. Llado L, Virgili J, Figueras J, et al. A prognostic index of the survival of patients with unresectable hepatocellular carcinoma after transcatheter arterial chemoembolization. *Cancer* 2000;88:50–57.

84. A comparison of lipiodol chemoembolization and conservative treatment for unresectable hepatocellular carcinoma. Groupe d'Etude et de Traitement du Carcinome Hépatocellulaire. *N Engl J Med* 1995;332:1256–1261.

85. Kulik LM, Carr BI, Mulcahy MF, et al. Safety and efficacy of 90Y radiotherapy for hepatocellular carcinoma with and without portal vein thrombosis. *Hepatology* 2008;47:71–81.

86. Georgiades CS, Hong K, D'Angelo M, et al. Safety and efficacy of transarterial chemoembolization in patients with unresectable hepatocellular carcinoma and portal vein thrombosis. *J Vasc Interv Radiol* 2005;16:1653.

87. Bruix J, Sala M, Llovet JM, et al. Chemoembolization for hepatocellular carcinoma. *Gastroenterology* 2004;127(Suppl): S179–S188.

88. Marelli L, Stigliano R, Triantos C, et al. Transarterial therapy for hepatocellular carcinoma: which technique is more effective? A systematic review of cohort and randomized studies. *Cardiovasc Intervent Radiol* 2007;30:6–25.

89. Schwarz RE, Abou-Alfa GK, Geschwind JF, et al. Nonoperative therapies for combined modality treatment of hepatocellular cancer: expert consensus statement. *HPB* 2010;5:313–320.

90. Lo CM, Ngan H, Tso WK, et al. Randomized controlled trial of transarterial lipiodol chemoembolization for unresectable hepatocellular carcinoma. *Hepatology* 2002;35:1164–1171.

91. Llovet JM, Real MI, Montana X, et al. Arterial embolisation or chemoembolisation versus symptomatic treatment in patients with unresectable hepatocellular carcinoma: a randomised controlled trial. *Lancet* 2002;359:1734–1749.

92. Llovet JM, Bruix J. Systematic review of randomized trials for unresectable hepatocellular carcinoma: chemoembolization improves survival. *Hepatology* 2003;37:429–442.

93. Millonig G, Graziadei W, Freund MC, et al. Response to preoperative chemoembolization correlates with outcome after liver transplantation in patients with hepatocellular carcinoma. *Liver Transpl* 2007;13:272–279.

94. Camma C, Schepis F, Orlando A, et al. Transarterial chemoembolization for unresectable hepatocellular carcinoma: meta-analysis of randomized controlled trials. *Radiology* 2002;224:47–54.

95. Lee KT, Lu YW, Wang SN, et al. The effect of preoperative transarterial chemoembolization of resectable hepatocellular carcinoma on clinical and economic outcomes. *J Surg Oncol* 2009;99:343–350.

96. Wu CC, Ho WZ, Ho WY, et al. Preoperative transcatheter arterial chemoembolization for resectable large hepatocellular carcinoma: a reappraisal. *Br J Surg* 1995;82:122–126.

97. Chan AO, Yuen MF, Hui CK, et al. A prospective study regarding the complications of transcatheter intraarterial lipiodol chemoembolization in patients with hepatocellular carcinoma. *Cancer* 2002;9:1747–1752.

98. Hong K, Khwaja J, Liapi E, et al. New intra-arterial drug delivery system for the treatment of liver cancer: preclinical assessment in a rabbit model of liver cancer. *Clin Cancer Res* 2006;12:2563–2567.

99. Lammer J, Malagari K, Vogl T, et al. Prospective randomized study of doxorubicin-eluting-bead embolization in the treatment of hepatocellular carcinoma: results of the PRECISION V study. *Cardiovasc Intervent Radiol* 2010;33: 41–52.

100. Dhanasekaran R, Kooby DA, Staley CA, et al. Comparison of conventional transarterial chemoembolization (TACE) and chemoembolization with doxorubicin drug eluting beads (DEB) for unresectable hepatocellular carcinoma (HCC). *J Surg Oncol* 2010;101:476–480.

101. Lewis AL, Gonzalez MV, Lloyd AW, et al. DC bead: in vitro characterization of a drug-delivery device for transarterial chemoembolization. *J Vasc Interv Radiol* 2006;17:335–342.

102. Maluccio MA, Covey AM, Porat LB, et al. Transcatheter arterial embolization with only particles for the treatment of unresectable hepatocellular carcinoma. *J Vasc Interv Radiol* 2008;19:862–869.

103. Bruix J, Llovet J, Castells A, et al. Transarterial embolization versus symptomatic treatment in patients with advanced hepatocellular carcinoma: results of a randomized, controlled trial in a single institution. *Hepatology* 1998;27:1578–1583.

104. Hawkins MA, Dawson LA. Radiation therapy for hepatocellular carcinoma: from palliation to cure. *Cancer* 2006;106: 1653–1663.

105. Salem R, Lewandowski RJ, Mulcahy MF, et al. Radioembolization for hepatocellular carcinoma using yttrium-90 microspheres: a comprehensive report of long-term outcomes. *Gastroenterology* 2010;138:52–64.

106. Sangro B, Carpanese L, Cianni R, et al. European multicenter evaluation of survival for patients with hepatocellular carcinoma (HCC) treated by radioembolization with ^{90}Y-labeled resin microspheres [abstract]. *J Clin Oncol* 2010; 28(Suppl 15s):4027.

107. Inarrairaegui M, Thurston KG, Bilbao JI, et al. Radioembolization with use of yttrium-90 resin microspheres in patients with hepatocellular carcinoma and portal vein thrombosis. *J Vasc Interv Radiol* 2010;21:1205–1212.

108. Tse RV, Hawkins M, Lockwood G, et al. Phase I study of individualized stereotactic body radiotherapy for hepatocellular carcinoma and intrahepatic cholangiocarcinoma. *J Clin Oncol* 2008;26:657–664.

109. Chiba T, Tokuuye K, Matsuzaki Y, et al. Proton beam therapy for hepatocellular carcinoma: a retrospective review of 162 patients. *Clin Cancer Res* 2005;11:3799–3805.

110. Hata M, Tokuuye K, Sugahara S, et al. Proton beam therapy for hepatocellular carcinoma with portal vein tumor thrombus. *Cancer* 2005;104:794–801.

111. Dawson LA. Protons or photons for hepatocellular carcinoma? Let's move forward together. *Int J Radiat Oncol Biol Phys* 2009;74:661–663.

112. Sandroussi C, Dawson LA, Lee M, et al. Radiotherapy as a bridge to liver transplantation for hepatocellular carcinoma. *Transpl Int* 2010;23:299–306.

113. Huang CC, Wu MC, Xu GW, et al. Overexpression of the MDR1 gene and P-glycoprotein in human hepatocellular carcinoma. *J Natl Cancer Inst* 1992;84:262–264.

114. Olweny CL, Toya T, Katongole-Mbidde E, et al. Treatment of hepatocellular carcinoma with Adriamycin. Preliminary communication. *Cancer* 1975;36:1250–1257.

115. Nerenstone SR, Ihde DC, Friedman MA, et al. Clinical trials in primary hepatocellular carcinoma: current status and future directions. *Cancer Treat Rev* 1988;15:1–31.

116. Mathurin P, Rixe O, Carbonell N, et al. Review article: overview of medical treatments in unresectable hepatocellular carcinoma—an impossible meta-analysis? *Aliment Pharmacol Ther* 1998;12:111–126.

117. Leung TW, Johnson PJ. Systemic therapy for hepatocellular carcinoma. *Semin Oncol* 2001;28:514–520.

118. Yang TS, Lin YC, Chen JS, et al. Phase II study of gemcitabine in patients with advanced hepatocellular carcinoma. *Cancer* 2000;89:750–756.
119. Porta C, Moroni M, Nastasi G, et al. 5-Fluorouracil and d, l-leucovorin calcium are active to treat unresectable hepatocellular carcinoma patients: preliminary results of a phase II study. *Oncology* 1995;52:487–491.
120. Patt YZ, Hassan MM, Aguayo A, et al. Oral capecitabine for the treatment of hepatocellular carcinoma, cholangiocarcinoma, and gallbladder carcinoma. *Cancer* 2004;101: 578–586.
121. O'Reilly EM, Stuart KE, Sanz-Altamira PM, et al. A phase II study of irinotecan in patients with advanced hepatocellular carcinoma. *Cancer* 2001;91:101–105.
122. Czauderna P, Mackinlay G, Perilongo G, et al. Hepatocellular carcinoma in children: results of the first prospective study of the International Society of Pediatric Oncology group. *J Clin Oncol* 2002;20:2798–2804.
123. Rai K, Tsuji A, Morita S, et al. Continuous infusion of 5-FU and low-dose consecutive CDDP therapy in advanced hepatocellular carcinoma: a phase II study [abstract]. *Proc Am Soc Clin Oncol* 2002;21:164a.
124. Louafi S, Boige V, Ducreux M, et al. Gemcitabine plus oxaliplatin (GEMOX) in patients with advanced hepatocellular carcinoma (HCC): results of a phase II study. *Cancer* 2007;109:1384–1390.
125. Leung TW, Patt YZ, Lau WY, et al. Complete pathological remission is possible with systemic combination chemotherapy for inoperable hepatocellular carcinoma. *Clin Cancer Res* 1999;5:1676–1681.
126. Yeo W, Mok TS, Zee B, et al. A randomized phase III study of doxorubicin versus cisplatin/interferon alpha-2b/doxorubicin/fluorouracil (PIAF) combination chemotherapy for unresectable hepatocellular carcinoma. *J Natl Cancer Inst* 2005;97:1532–1538.
127. Villa E, Colantoni A, Grottola A, et al. Variant estrogen receptors and their role in liver disease. *Mol Cell Endocrinol* 2002;193:65–69.
128. Nowak A, Findlay M, Culjak G, et al. Tamoxifen for hepatocellular carcinoma. *Cochrane Database Syst Rev* 2004;3: CD001024.
129. Verhoef C, van Dekken H, Hofland LJ, et al. Somatostatin receptor in human hepatocellular carcinomas: biological, patient and tumor characteristics. *Dig Surg* 2008;25:21–26.
130. Guo TK, Hao XY, Ma B, et al. Octreotide for advanced hepatocellular carcinoma: a meta-analysis of randomized controlled trials. *J Cancer Res Clin Oncol* 2009;135:1685–1692.

131. Liu L, Cao Y, Chen C, et al. Sorafenib blocks the RAF/MEK/ERK pathway, inhibits tumor angiogenesis, and induces tumor cell apoptosis in hepatocellular carcinoma model PLC/PRF/5. *Cancer Res* 2006;66:11851–11858.

132. Abou-Alfa GK, Schwartz L, Ricci S, et al. Phase II study of sorafenib in patients with advanced hepatocellular carcinoma. *J Clin Oncol* 2006;24:4293–4300.

133. Llovet JM, Ricci S, Mazzaferro V, et al. Sorafenib in advanced hepatocellular carcinoma. *N Engl J Med* 2008;359:378–390.

134. Cheng AL, Kang YK, Chen Z, et al. Efficacy and safety of sorafenib in patients in the Asia-Pacific region with advanced hepatocellular carcinoma: a phase III randomised, double-blind, placebo-controlled trial. *Lancet Oncol* 2009;10:25–34.

135. Huitzil FD, Saltz LS, Song J, et al. Retrospective analysis of outcome in hepatocellular carcinoma (HCC) patients (pts) with hepatitis C (C+) versus B (B+) treated with sorafenib (S). Program and abstracts of the 2008 Gastrointestinal Cancers Symposium, January 19-21, 2008, Orlando, FL, Abstract 173.

136. Bolondi L, Caspary W, Bennouna J, et al. Clinical benefit of sorafenib in hepatitis C patients with hepatocellular carcinoma (HCC): subgroup analysis of the SHARP trial. 2008 Gastrointestinal Cancers Symposium, Orlando, FL, Abstract 129.

137. Abou-Alfa GK, Amadori D, Santoro A, et al. Is sorafenib (S) safe and effective in patients (pts) with hepatocellular carcinoma (HCC) and Child-Pugh B (CPB) cirrhosis? *J Clin Oncol* 2008;26(Suppl):217s.

138. Pinter M, Sieghart W, Graziadei I, et al. Sorafenib in unresectable hepatocellular carcinoma from mild to advanced stage liver cirrhosis. *Oncologist* 2009;14:70–76.

139. Yau T, Chan P, Ng K, et al. Efficacy and tolerability of single agent sorafenib in poor risk advanced hepatocellular carcinoma patients. *J Clin Oncol* 2008;26(Suppl):15513.

140. Miller AA, Murry DJ, Owzar K, et al. Phase I and pharmacokinetic study of sorafenib in patients with hepatic or renal dysfunction: CALGB 60301. *J Clin Oncol* 2009;27:1800–1805.

141. Abou-Alfa GK, Johnson P, Knox JJ, et al. Doxorubicin plus sorafenib vs doxorubicin alone in patients with advanced hepatocellular carcinoma: a randomized trial. *JAMA* 2010;304:2154–2160.

142. Okita K, Imanaka K, Chida W, et al. Phase III study of sorafenib in patients in Japan and Korea with advanced hepatocellular carcinoma (HCC) treated after transarterial chemoembolization (TACE). 2010 Gastrointestinal Cancers Symposium, Orlando, FL, Abstract LBA128.

143. El-Khoueiry AB. Education session: update on gastrointestinal noncolorectal malignancies: what's new since the 2009

ASCO Annual Meeting? Hepatobiliary and pancreatic cancers since ASCO 2009: steady steps forward and a long way to go. Gastrointestinal (noncolorectal) Cancer Track, 2010 ASCO Annual Meeting, June 4–8, 2010, Chicago, IL.

144. Philip PA, Mahoney MR, Allmer C, et al. Phase II study of erlotinib (OSI-774) in patients with advanced hepatocellular cancer. *J Clin Oncol* 2005;23:6657–6663.

145. Pawlik TM, Reyes DK, Cosgrove D, et al. Phase II trial of sorafenib combined with concurrent transarterial chemoembolization with doxorubicin-eluting beads for hepatocellular carcinoma. *J Clin Oncol* 2011.

146. Ramanathan RK, Belani CP, Singh DA, et al. A phase II study of lapatinib in patients with advanced biliary tree and hepatocellular cancer. *Cancer Chemother Pharmacol* 2009;64:777–783.

147. Gruenwald V, Wilkens L, Gebel M, et al. A phase II open-label study of cetuximab in unresectable hepatocellular carcinoma: final results. *J Clin Oncol* 2007;25(Suppl 18S):4598.

148. Zhu AX, Stuart K, Blaszkowsky LS, et al. Phase 2 study of cetuximab in patients with advanced hepatocellular carcinoma. *Cancer* 2007;110:581–589.

149. Desbois-Mouthon C, Baron A, Blivet-Van Eggelpoël MJ, et al. Insulin-like growth factor-1 receptor inhibition induces a resistance mechanism via the epidermal growth factor receptor/HER3/AKT signaling pathway: rational basis for co-targeting insulin-like growth factor-1 receptor and epidermal growth factor receptor in hepatocellular carcinoma. *Clin Cancer Res* 2009;15:5445–5456.

150. Wang SY, Chen B, Zhan YQ, et al. SU5416 is a potent inhibitor of hepatocyte growth factor receptor (c-Met) and blocks HGF-induced invasiveness of human HepG2 hepatoma cells. *J Hepatol* 2004;41:267–273.

151. Borbath I, Santoro A, Van Laetham J, et al. ARQ 197–215: a randomized, placebo-controlled phase II clinical trial evaluating the c-Met inhibitor, ARQ 197, in patients (pts) with hepatocellular carcinoma (HCC). *J Clin Oncol* 2010;28 (Suppl 15s):TPS215.

152. Siegel AB, Cohen EI, Ocean A, et al. Phase II trial evaluating the clinical and biologic effects of bevacizumab in unresectable hepatocellular carcinoma. *J Clin Oncol* 2008;26:2992–2998.

153. Malka D, Dromain C, Farace F, et al. Bevacizumab in patients (pts) with advanced hepatocellular carcinoma (HCC): preliminary results of a phase II study with circulating endothelial cell (CEC) monitoring. *J Clin Oncol* 2007;25(Suppl 18S):4570.

154. Zhu AX, Blaszkowsky LS, Ryan DP, et al. Phase II study of gemcitabine and oxaliplatin in combination with bevacizumab in patients with advanced hepatocellular carcinoma. *J Clin Oncol* 2006;24:1898–1903.

155. Hsu CH, Yang TS, Hsu C, et al. Efficacy and tolerability of bevacizumab plus capecitabine as first-line therapy in patients with advanced hepatocellular carcinoma. *Br J Cancer* 2010;102:981–986.

156. Sun W, Haller DG, Mykulowycz K, et al. Combination of capecitabine, oxaliplatin with bevacizumab in treatment of advanced hepatocellular carcinoma (HCC): a phase II study. *J Clin Oncol* 2007;25(Suppl 18S):4574.

157. Thomas MB, Morris JS, Chadha R, et al. Phase II trial of the combination of bevacizumab and erlotinib in patients who have advanced hepatocellular carcinoma. *J Clin Oncol* 2009;27:843–850.

158. Schwartz JD, Schwartz M, Lehrer D, et al. Bevacizumab in unresectable hepatocellular carcinoma (HCC) for patients without metastasis and without invasion of the portal vein. *J Clin Oncol* 2006;24(Suppl 18S):4144.

159. Faivre S, Raymond E, Boucher E, et al. Safety and efficacy of sunitinib in patients with advanced hepatocellular carcinoma: an open-label, multicentre, phase II study. *Lancet Oncol* 2009;10:794–800.

160. Zhu AX, Sahani DV, Duda DG, et al. Efficacy, safety, and potential biomarkers of sunitinib monotherapy in advanced hepatocellular carcinoma: a phase II study. *J Clin Oncol* 2009;27:3027–3035.

161. Cheng A, Kang Y, Lin D et al. Phase III trial of sunitinib (Su) versus sorafenib (So) in advanced hepatocellular carcinoma (HCC). *J Clin Oncol* 2011;29(Suppl, abstract 4000).

162. Toh H, Chen P, Carr BI, et al. Linifanib phase II trial in patients with advanced hepatocellular carcinoma (HCC). *J Clin Oncol* 2010;28(Suppl 15s):4038.

163. Raoul JL, Finn RS, Kang YK, et al. An open-label phase II study of first- and second-line treatment with brivanib in patients with hepatocellular carcinoma (HCC). *J Clin Oncol* 2009;27(Suppl 15s):4577.

164. Kato K, Cox AD, Hisaka MM, et al. Isoprenoid addition to Ras protein is the critical modification for its membrane association and transforming activity. *Proceedings of the National Academy of Sciences of the United States of America.* 1992:89(14):6403–6407.

165. Goldstein JL, Brown MS. Regulation of the mevalonate pathway. *Nature* 1990:343(6257):425–430.

166. Toso S, Merani S, Bigam DL, et al. Sirolimus-based immunosuppression is associated with increased survival after liver transplantation for hepatocellular carcinoma. *Hepatology* 2010;51:1237–1243.

167. Zimmerman MA, Trotter JF, Wachs M, et al. Sirolimus-based immunosuppression following liver transplantation for hepatocellular carcinoma. *Liver Transpl* 2008;14:633–638.

168. Chen YB, Sun YA, Gong JP. Effects of rapamycin in liver transplantation. *Hepatobiliary Pancreas Dis Int* 2008;7:25–28.
169. Zhou J, Fan J, Wang Z, et al. Conversion to sirolimus immunosuppression in liver transplantation recipients with hepatocellular carcinoma: report of an initial experience. *World J Gastroenterol* 2006;12:3114–3118.
170. Abou-Alfa GK, Zhao B, Capanu M, et al. Tumor necrosis as a correlate for response in subgroup of patients with advanced hepatocellular carcinoma (HCC) treated with sorafenib. ESMO 2008, Stockholm, Sweden, Abstract 547P.
171. Lencioni R, Llovet JM. Modified RECIST (mRECIST) assessment for hepatocellular carcinoma. *Semin Liver Dis* 2010;30:52–60.
172. Bruix J, Sherman M, Llovet JM, et al. Clinical management of hepatocellular carcinoma. Conclusions of the Barcelona-2000 EASL conference. European Association for the Study of the Liver. *J Hepatol* 2001;35:421–430.
173. Sala M, Llovet JM, Vilana R, et al. Barcelona Clinic Liver Cancer Group. Initial response to percutaneous ablation predicts survival in patients with hepatocellular carcinoma. *Hepatology* 2004;40:1352–1360.
174. Riaz A, Miller FH, Kulik LM, et al. Imaging response in the primary index lesion and clinical outcomes following transarterial locoregional therapy for hepatocellular carcinoma. *JAMA* 2010;303:1062–1069.
175. Yeo W, Chan PKS, Zhong S, et al. Frequency of hepatitis B virus reactivation in cancer patients undergoing cytotoxic chemotherapy: a prospective study of 626 patients with identification of risk factors. *J Med Virol* 2000;62:299–307.
176. Alexopoulos CG, Vaslamatzis M, Hatzidimitriou G. Prevalence of hepatitis B virus marker positivity and evolution of hepatitis B virus profile, during chemotherapy, in patients with solid tumours. *Br J Cancer* 1999;81:69–74.
177. Yeo W, Lam KC, Zee B, et al. Hepatitis C reactivation in patients with hepatocellular carcinoma undergoing systemic chemotherapy. *Ann Oncol* 2004;15:1661–1666.
178. Mendelsohn RB, Nagula S, Taur Y, et al. Reactivation of chronic hepatitis B virus in cancer patients receiving immunosuppression: the case for screening. *J Clin Oncol* 2010; 28(Suppl 15s):9088.
179. Yeo W, Mo FK, Chan SL, et al. Hepatitis B viral load predicts survival of HCC patients undergoing systemic chemotherapy. *Hepatology* 2007;45:1382–1389.
180. Ludwig E, Mendelsohn RB, Taur Y, et al. Prevalence of hepatitis B surface antigen and hepatitis B core antibody in a population initiating immunosuppressive therapy. *J Clin Oncol* 2010;28(Suppl 15s):9009.

181. de Pree C, Giostra E, Galetto A, et al. Hepatitis C virus acute exacerbation during chemotherapy and radiotherapy for esophageal carcinoma. *Ann Oncol* 1994;5:861–862.

182. Santini D, Picardi A, Vincenzi B, et al. Severe liver dysfunction after raltitrexed administration in an HCV-positive colorectal cancer patient. *Cancer Invest* 2003;21:162–163.

183. Melisko ME, Fox R, Venook A. Reactivation of hepatitis C virus after chemotherapy for colon cancer. *Clin Oncol* 2004; 16:204–205.

184. Vento S, Cainelli F, Mirandola F, et al. Fulminant hepatitis on withdrawal of chemotherapy in carriers of hepatitis C virus. *Lancet* 1996;347:92–93.

185. Jarnagin W, Chapman WC, Curley S, et al. Surgical treatment of hepatocellular carcinoma: expert consensus statement. *HPB* 2010;12:302–310.

186. Wang J, Wang F, Kessinger A. Outcome of combined hepatocellular and cholangiocarcinoma of the liver. *J Oncol* 2010;2010:917356.

187. Chan AC, Lo CM, Ng IO, et al. Liver transplantation for combined hepatocellular cholangiocarcinoma. *Asian J Surg* 2007;30:143–146.

188. Dick EA, Taylor-Robinson SD, Thomas HC, et al. Ablative therapy for liver tumors. *Gut* 2002;50:733–739.

CHAPTER 8

Surveillance, Screening, and Prevention

■ Surveillance

- Surveillance refers to the use of screening investigations among individuals at increased risk for developing a particular disease with the objective of decreasing disease-specific mortality.[1]
- Despite the strong rationale for implementing standardized screening programs for at-risk individuals, the issue of whether screening reduces hepatocellular carcinoma (HCC) mortality has not been definitively established.[2] Data are conflicting with respect to the cost-effectiveness and sensitivity of screening at detecting disease when it is potentially curable.[3–5]
- Support for screening has mainly been derived from observational and uncontrolled series suggesting a benefit, particularly among those infected with viral hepatitis.[5–9] However, the low incidence of HCC among those with non-viral hepatitis–induced cirrhosis has made it difficult to determine the degree of benefit in these patients.
- A randomized controlled trial that specifically address the mortality benefit of screening was conducted in Shanghai, China.[7]
  - In the study, 18,816 patients with hepatitis B virus (HBV) infection or chronic hepatitis were randomized to screening with serum α-fetoprotein (AFP) levels and liver ultrasonography biannually compared to no screening.
  - Despite a compliance rate of only 58.2% among individuals assigned to the screening arm, HCC mortality was reduced by 37%.

- The applicability of this study's findings to patients with other causes of chronic liver disease is unclear. For practical purposes, however, screening is recommended for at-risk patients, as will be discussed below (**Table 8.1**).

■ Who Should Be Screened?

American Association for the Study of Liver Disease (AASLD) Recommendations[10]

- Asian HBV carriers without cirrhosis should be screened beginning at age 40 if male or at age 50 if female.
  - The annual incidence of HCC in these patients is 0.3–0.6%.[11,12]
  - Even those without serum HBV surface antigens (i.e., sero-clearance) as a result of treatment or spontaneous clearance remain at risk and should continue long-term screening.[13]
  - Caucasian HBV carriers without cirrhosis or active viral replication have a low risk of developing HCC, and the benefit of screening this population is less clear.[14,15]
- HBV carriers with a family history of HCC should be screened.
- African blacks with HBV have been reported to develop HCC within the fourth decade of life and should begin screening at a younger age, although the age threshold has not been specified.[16,17]
- All individuals with HBV or hepatitis C virus (HCV) cirrhosis should begin screening upon diagnosis. The annual HCC incidence in this population is 2–8%.
  - Although sero-clearance following treatment probably decreases the risk of developing HCC, the risk does not disappear, and patients should continue to undergo screening.
- Patients coinfected with HIV and viral hepatitis who develop HCC tend to have more aggressive disease[18] that is less likely to be amenable to therapy at presentation. Nevertheless, these patients appear to benefit from the same screening procedures recommended for patients infected with viral hepatitis and should be followed accordingly.[19]

▪ Patients with stage IV primary biliary cirrhosis (PBC) should be screened.
  • The incidence and prevalence of HCC in patients with stage III/IV PBC ranges from 3–6%.[20,21]
  • Independent risk factors for the development of HCC include male sex, age > 70 years, a history of blood transfusions, and clinical evidence of ascites, portal hypertension, or cirrhosis.[22]
▪ Patients with metabolic causes of cirrhosis (i.e., hereditary hemochromatosis, α-1-antitrypsin deficiency, alcohol, nonalcoholic fatty liver disease, autoimmune) should be screened.
  • The benefit of surveillance in patients with nonalcoholic fatty liver disease *without* cirrhosis is unclear.
▪ Although the presence of an elevated AFP,[23] regenerative nodules,[24,25] dysplasia,[26] increased hepatocyte proliferative indices,[27,28] and high HBV viral load[29] are associated with a more imminent risk of developing HCC, patients with these features should continue screening at the standard schedule.

National Comprehensive Cancer Network (NCCN) Guidelines[30]

▪ HBV carriers without cirrhosis, including patients with active viral replication, high HBV DNA levels, a family history of HCC, Asian patients ($\geq$ 40 years if male, $\geq$ 50 years if female), and African patients $\geq$ 20 years old, should be screened.
▪ Patients should be screened if they have cirrhosis due to viral hepatitis, alcohol, autoimmune hepatitis, hemochromatosis, α-1-antitrypsin deficiency, primary biliary cirrhosis, and nonalcoholic steatohepatitis.

▪ How Should Surveillance Be Performed?

AASLD Guidelines

▪ Abdominal ultrasonography should be performed every 6 months in at-risk patients.[10]
▪ Serum AFP has insufficient sensitivity and specificity for HCC screening.[31] It should not be used in isolation for surveillance unless ultrasonography is unavailable.[32]

Table 8.1   Patients Who Should Undergo Surveillance for HCC

Hepatitis B virus (HBV) infection
    Asian carriers without cirrhosis; begin at age 40 for male, age 50 for
    female
    African black carriers without cirrhosis ≥ 20 years
    Carrier, noncirrhotic with a family history of HCC
    Carrier, noncirrhotic with serologic evidence of active replication
    Carrier, noncirrhotic with high HBV DNA level
    All carriers with cirrhosis

Hepatitis C virus infection
    All carriers with cirrhosis

Patients coinfected with HIV and viral hepatitis

Stage IV primary biliary cirrhosis

**Metabolic and inherited causes of chronic liver disease with
cirrhosis**
    Nonalcoholic steatohepatitis
    Alcohol
    Autoimmune hepatitis
    Hereditary hemochromatosis
    Alpha-1-antitrypsin deficiency

- There is no basis for alternating between ultrasound and serum AFP.[10] Combined serologic and radiologic testing increases the detection rate, but is more expensive and leads to more false-positives results.[33]
- The surveillance interval does not need to be shortened for individuals with high-risk clinical or histologic features (e.g., co-infection with human immunodeficiency virus [HIV], increased AFP, dysplasia, high proliferative index or viral load).[10]

NCCN Guidelines[30]

- In general, the NCCN recommendations for HCC screening are similar to those of the AASLD.
- Patients considered to be at risk for developing HCC should undergo screening with an abdominal ultrasound and serum AFP every 6–12 months.

- Although the NCCN guidelines acknowledge the limitations of serum AFP levels, serial measurements every 6 months are still recommended as an adjunct given the operator dependence of ultrasonography.[30]

■ Recall Policies: What to Do if a Screening Test Result Is Abnormal

- Any new nodule not seen on a prior screening ultrasound or a nodule that is growing over time even if previously considered benign is considered abnormal and warrants further investigation.[1]
- The AASLD recommends an algorithmic approach to the appropriate management of a suspicious liver nodule. The decision to biopsy or monitor a lesion depends on its size, radiographic contrast enhancement pattern, and serum AFP levels. This is outlined further in Chapter 3: Diagnostic Workup.
- The NCCN guidelines generally follow the AASLD algorithm. An exception is that the presence of a rising AFP warrants further imaging with a triphasic computed tomography (CT) or magnetic resonance imaging (MRI) scan to determine whether a mass is present. Positron emission tomography (PET)-CT scans are considered a suboptimal imaging modality. If a mass is found, subsequent investigations and management are as for HCC. If no mass is found, surveillance should continue with an ultrasound and serum AFP every 3 months.[30]

■ Prevention of HCC

- Primary prevention of HCC consists of avoidance of alcohol and other known hepatotoxins and hepatocarcinogens.
- Hepatocellular adenomas are benign lesions that usually occur in women of reproductive age who use oral contraceptives,[34] although they have also been reported in men taking anabolic steroids.[35] These lesions have malignant potential, and surgical resection is an effective preventative measure.[36]
- High-grade dysplastic nodules (H-DNs) are premalignant lesions that evolve into HCC in 35% of patients.[37] Surgical

resection or locoregional ablative therapies such as percutaneous microwave ablation[38] may be considered for primary prevention of HCC in patients with adequate liver function.

- Early detection and phlebotomy in patients with hereditary hemochromatosis may prevent or even reverse the development of cirrhosis.[39,40] This, in turn, could prevent the development of HCC, but the risk still exists.[40,41]

- Acyclic retinoids are vitamin A analogs that have shown promise for the secondary prevention of recurrent HCC in patients who have undergone curative surgery or percutaneous ethanol injection.[42] However, this approach remains investigational.

■ References

1. Hodgson DC, Tannock IF. Guide to studies of diagnostic tests, prognostic factors, and treatments. In: Tannock IF, Hill R, Bristow R, et al (eds). *Basic Science of Oncology*. Toronto: McGraw-Hill Medical Publishing Division, 2005:485–507.

2. De Masi S Tosti ME, Mele A. Screening for hepatocellular carcinoma. *Dig Liver Dis* 2005;37:260–268.

3. Bolondi L, Sofia S, Siringo S, et al. Surveillance programme of cirrhotic patients for early diagnosis and treatment of hepatocellular carcinoma: a cost effectiveness analysis. *Gut* 2001;48:251–259.

4. Patel D, Terreault NA, Yao FY, et al. Cost-effectiveness of hepatocellular carcinoma surveillance in patients with hepatitis C virus-related cirrhosis. *Clin Gastroenterol Hepatol* 2005;3:75–84.

5. Leykum LK, El-Serag HB, Cornell J, et al. Screening for hepatocellular carcinoma among veterans with hepatitis C on disease stage, treatment received, and survival. *Clin Gastroenterol Hepatol* 2007;5:508–512.

6. McMahon BJ, Bulkow L, Harpster A, et al. Screening for hepatocellular carcinoma in Alaska natives infected with chronic hepatitis B: a 16-year population-based study. *Hepatology* 2000;32:842–846.

7. Wun YT, Dickinson JA. Alpha-fetoprotein and/or liver ultrasonography for liver cancer screening in patients with chronic hepatitis B. *Cochrane Database Syst Rev* 2003;2:CD002799.

8. Stravitz RT, Heuman DM, Chand N, et al. Surveillance for hepatocellular carcinoma in patients with cirrhosis improves outcome. *Am J Med* 2008;121:119–126.

9. Zhang BH, Yang BH, Tang ZY. Randomized controlled trial of screening for hepatocellular carcinoma. *J Cancer Res Clin Oncol* 2004;130:417–422.

10. Bruix J, Sherman M. AASLD practice guideline. Management of hepatocellular carcinoma: an update. *Hepatology* 2011;53:1020–1022.

11. Beasley RP, Hwang LY, Lin CC, et al. Hepatocellular carcinoma and hepatitis B virus. A prospective study of 22 707 men in Taiwan. *Lancet* 1981;2:1129–1133.

12. Sakuma K, Saitoh N, Kasai M, et al. Relative risks of death due to liver disease among Japanese male adults having various statuses for hepatitis B s and e antigen/antibody in serum: a prospective study. *Hepatology* 1988;8:1642–1646.

13. Yuen MF, Wong DK, Sablon E, et al. HBsAg seroclearance in chronic hepatitis B in the Chinese: virological, histological, and clinical aspects. *Hepatology* 2004;39:1694–1701.

14. de Franchis R, Meucchi G, Vecchi M, et al. The natural history of asymptomatic hepatitis B surface antigen carriers. *Ann Intern Med* 1993;118:191–194.

15. Fattovich G. Natural history of hepatitis B. *J Hepatol* 2003; 39(Suppl 1):S50–S58.

16. Kew MC, Marcus R, Geddes EW. Some characteristics of Mozambican Shangaans with primary hepatocellular carcinoma. *S Afr Med J* 1977;51:306–309.

17. Kew MC, Macerollo P. Effect of age on the etiologic role of hepatitis B infection in hepatocellular carcinoma in blacks. *Gastroenterology* 1988;94:439–442.

18. Rosenthal E, Poiree M, Pradier C, et al. Mortality due to hepatitis C-related liver disease in HIV-infected patients in France (Mortavic 2001 study). *Aids* 2003;17:1803–1809.

19. Kikuchi L, Nunez M, Barreiro P, et al; Liver Cancer in HIV Study Group. Impact of screening for hepatocellular carcinoma (HCC) in HIV/HCV-coinfected patients on staging, therapy and survival. 45th Annual Meeting of the European Association for the Study of the Liver (EASL 2010), Vienna, Austria, April 14–18, 2010.

20. Jones DE, Metcalf JV, Collier JD, et al. Hepatocellular carcinoma in primary biliary cirrhosis and its impact on outcomes. *Hepatology* 1997;26:1138–1142.

21. Cavazza A, Caballeria L, Floreani A, et al. Incidence, risk factors, and survival of hepatocellular carcinoma in primary biliary cirrhosis: comparative analysis from two centers. *Hepatology* 2009;50:1162–1168.

22. Suzuki A, Lymp J, Donlinger J, et al. Clinical predictors for hepatocellular carcinoma in patients with primary biliary cirrhosis. *Clin Gastroenterol Hepatol* 2007;5:259–264.

23. Oka H, Tamori A, Kuroki T, et al. Prospective study of alpha-fetoprotein in cirrhotic patients monitored for development of hepatocellular carcinoma. *Hepatology* 1994;19:61–66.

24. Hytiroglou P, Theise ND, Schwartz M, et al. Macroregenerative nodules in a series of adult cirrhotic liver explants: issues

of classification and nomenclature. *Hepatology* 1995;21: 703–708.

25. Shibata M, Morizane T, Uchida T, et al. Irregular regeneration of hepatocytes and risk of hepatocellular carcinoma in chronic hepatitis and cirrhosis with hepatitis C virus infection. *Lancet* 1998;351:1773–1777.

26. Lee RG, Tsamandas AC, Demetris AJ. Large cell change (liver cell dysplasia) and hepatocellular carcinoma in cirrhosis: matched case control study, pathological analysis, and pathogenetic hypothesis. *Hepatology* 1997;26:1415–1422.

27. Donato MF, Arosio E, Del Ninno E, et al. High rates of hepatocellular carcinoma in cirrhotic patients with high liver cell proliferative activity. *Hepatology* 2001;34:523–528.

28. Borzio M, Trere D, Borzio F, et al. Hepatocyte proliferation rate is a powerful parameter for predicting hepatocellular carcinoma development in liver cirrhosis. *Mol Pathol* 1998; 51:96–101.

29. Chen CJ, Yang HI, Su J, et al. Risk of hepatocellular carcinoma across a biological gradient of serum hepatitis B virus DNA level. *JAMA* 2006;295:65–73.

30. National Comprehensive Cancer Network. Hepatobiliary cancers. NCCN Clinical Practice Guidelines. August 13, 2010. http://www.nccn.org/professionals/physician_gls/PDF/hepatobiliary.pdf.

31. Lok AS, Sterling RK, Everhart JE, et al. Des-gamma-carboxy prothrombin and alpha-fetoprotein as biomarkers for the early detection of hepatocellular carcinoma. *Gastroenterology* 2010;138:493–502.

32. Bruix J, Sherman M. Management of hepatocellular carcinoma. *Hepatology* 2005;42:1208–1236.

33. Zhang B, Yang B. Combined alpha fetoprotein testing and ultrasonography as a screening test for primary liver cancer. *J Med Screen* 1999;6:108–110.

34. Edmondson HA, Henderson B, Benton B. Liver cell adenomas associated with use of oral contraceptives. *N Engl J Med* 1976;294:470–472.

35. Bagia S, Hewitt PM, Morris DL. Anabolic steroid-induced hepatic adenomas with spontaneous haemorrhage in a bodybuilder. *Aust N Z J Surg* 2000;70:686–687.

36. van der Windt DJ, Kok NF, Hussain SM, et al. Case oriented approach to the management of hepatocellular adenoma. *Br J Surg* 2006;93:1495–1502.

37. Takayama T, Makuuchi M, Hirohashi S, et al. Malignant transformation of adenomatous hyperplasia to hepatocellular carcinoma. *Lancet* 1990;336:1150–1153.

38. Liang P, Dong B, Yu X, et al. Sonography-guided percutaneous microwave ablation of high-grade dysplastic nodules in cirrhotic liver. *AJR Am J Roentgenol* 2005;184:1657–1660.

39. Niederau C, Fischer R, Sonnenberg A, et al. Survival and causes of death in cirrhotic and non-cirrhotic patients with primary hemochromatosis. *N Engl J Med* 1985;313:1256–1262.
40. Blumberg RS, Chopra S, Ibrahim R, et al. Primary hepatocellular carcinoma in idiopathic hemochromatosis after reversal of cirrhosis. *Gastroenterology* 1988;95:1399–1402.
41. Singh P, Kaur H, Lerner RG, et al. Hepatocellular carcinoma in non-cirrhotic liver without evidence of iron overload in a patient with primary hemochromatosis. Review. *J Gastrointest Cancer* [Epub ahead of print on September 28, 2010].
42. Muto Y, Moriwaki H, Saito A. Prevention of second primary tumors by an acyclic retinoid in patients with hepatocellular carcinoma. *N Engl J Med* 1999;340:1046–1047.

CHAPTER 9

Future Trends and Controversies

■ Introduction

With new therapeutic options and strategies for screening and diagnosis available, the best way to integrate and use these tools in a safe, biologically sound, and clinically meaningful way is an ongoing learning curve.

■ Predictive and Prognostic Biomarkers

- In addition to developing therapeutic targets, the full elucidation of the genetic and molecular alterations underlying hepatocellular carcinoma (HCC) will hopefully identify predictive and prognostic biomarkers that can inform therapeutic choices and guide clinical decision making.

- Prognostic biomarkers provide information about the natural history of a disease independent of therapy. Candidates include *c-MET* overexpression,[1] mammalian target of rapamycin (*mTOR*) dysregulation,[2,3] *TP53* and *CDKN2A* mutations,[4–6] and low miR-26 expression levels,[7] all of which have been associated with poorer survival.

- A predictive biomarker provides information about how a patient might be expected to respond to therapy.
  - Infection with hepatitis C virus (HCV) upregulates one of the targets of sorafenib and has been associated with better survival on therapy, making it a potential predictive biomarker.[8–10]
  - Recently, sorafenib has been shown to suppress proangiogenic signaling by vascular endothelial growth factor (VEGF), platelet-derived growth factor (PDGF), and Raf kinase, in addition to normalizing splanchnic

circulation in mouse simulated models of portal hypertension and cirrhosis.[11] The value of using changes in the levels of proangiogenic factors as biomarkers of response to sorafenib in patients with HCC will potentially be explored in a multicenter clinical trial.[12]

■ All of these potential biomarkers will require prospective validation before they can be accepted as a part of standard clinical practice.

■ Managing Patients with HCC and Moderate-Severe Liver Dysfunction

■ Patients with HCC and Child-Pugh B or C liver dysfunction are a neglected population; concerns about excess toxicity often limit or preclude treatment, resulting in their exclusion from clinical trials. There is clearly a dearth of treatment options for these patients.

■ Retrospective studies of patients with Child-Pugh B/C or Child-Pugh A cirrhosis and portal vein thrombosis who were treated with sorafenib have reported grade 3/4 adverse events in 20–34% of patients, leading to dose reductions and treatment discontinuations in up to 78%, as well as shorter survival times.[13–16]

• The original phase II study of sorafenib in patients with both Child-Pugh A and B cirrhosis found that although the pharmacokinetic, toxicity, and drug discontinuation rates were similar, Child-Pugh B patients developed more hyperbilirubinemia and signs of hepatic decompensation on therapy.[16,17] Time to progression and overall survival were shorter for the Child-Pugh B patients, although it was unclear whether this was due to the shorter time on treatment or underlying disease biology.[16]

■ Although sorafenib can potentially still be given to patients with more severe hepatic dysfunction using lower doses and alternate dosing schedules,[13] this must be done cautiously and remains an area that requires further study in patients with HCC.

■ An important objective for trials investigating newer drugs for HCC will be to examine their efficacy and safety in patients with decreased liver function. Recently, a phase II trial of the antiangiogenic compound linifanib (ABT-869), reported inferior outcomes as well as one death due to an intracranial hemorrhage in the group of patients with Child-Pugh B cirrhosis.[18]

- Studies of patients with chronic liver disease have identified the following serum markers that appear to be associated with the development subsequent hepatic fibrosis: hyaluronic acid, amino-terminal propeptide of type III collagen, and tissue inhibitor of matrix metalloproteinase 1.[19] These markers might potentially be incorporated into studies of patients with HCC and severe liver disease as a means of monitoring for signs of impending liver failure and hopefully prevent its occurrence.[12]

■ Response Assessment Criteria in the Age of Biologic Therapies

- Response Evaluation Criteria in Solid Tumors (RECIST) guidelines, which measure changes in tumor dimensions, do not adequately capture responses to biologic therapies.
- In both of the phase III trials of sorafenib for advanced HCC, survival benefits were seen despite the relative absence of objective responses.[17,20]
- Investigators have looked at the ratio of tumor necrosis to tumor volume in patients treated with sorafenib and have found this to correlate significantly with response to sorafenib.[21,22]
- Modified RECIST guidelines include a decrease in intratumoral arterial enhancement among the criteria necessary to declare a response to antiangiogenic therapies like sorafenib.
- Advanced functional imaging studies such dynamic contrast-enhanced magnetic resonance imaging (DCE-MRI) have demonstrated decreases in arterial enhancement concurrent with decreases in circulating proangiogenic factors in patients treated with bevacizumab.[23]
  - In another study of patients who received doxorubicin and sorafenib, changes in vascular flow and permeability

assessed by DCE-MRI did not correlate significantly with responses.[24]

- Antiangiogenic agents themselves can alter tumor vasculature, producing the appearance of decreased enhancement without exerting any antitumoral effects.[25]

- The best imaging modalities and optimal response assessment parameters are clearly areas of controversy that warrant further investigation. Histopathologic confirmation of radiographic responses may prove necessary for validation.

■ Novel Therapeutic Approaches

- Biologic therapies targeting aberrant intracellular signaling pathways continue to be developed and tested. Agents like sorafenib that are active in the advanced setting are now being evaluated in the adjuvant setting following surgery, locoregional ablative therapies, or liver transplantation.

- Immunotherapy is another novel treatment strategy being explored in HCC.
  - Glypican-3 is a heparin sulfate proteoglycan found to be overexpressed on HCC cells with remarkable specificity.[26]
  - Preclinical trials have shown that embryonic stem cell–derived dendritic cells that express glypican-3 are able to induce a host immune response against melanoma in mice.[27]
  - GC33 is an anti–glypican-3 antibody shown to induce natural killer cell–mediated tumor destruction.[28] GC33 is currently being evaluated in combination with sorafenib in a phase I trial (ClinicalTrials.gov, NCT00976170).

■ Etiology-Based Treatment and Outcomes of HCC

- As discussed in previous chapters, the various etiologies and risk factors for liver damage exert their effects through different mechanisms that can interact and potentiate each other, culminating in the development of HCC. Furthermore, there is increasing evidence that the different etiologies are associated with different genetic aberrations and clinical outcomes.

- Compared to patients with hepatitis B virus (HBV) who go on to develop HCC, patients with HCV fare worse after surgery with respect to the risk of recurrence and disease-free survival.[29,30] This is likely due to the underlying cirrhosis and consequent impairment in hepatic reserve associated with HCV.
- HCV patients appear to have an improved outcome using sorafenib, when compared to HBV patients. This is based on very limited, only hypothesis-generating data and is possibly explained by the upregulation of Raf1, a target of sorafenib.[31]
- HBV has been shown to have a causal role in the upregulation of c-MET[32] and inactivation of p53,[33,34] both of which may have implications for prognosis.[1,35]
- Both doxorubicin and the direct thymidylate synthase inhibitor, nolatrexed, may have differential activity in HBV-predominant populations compared to mixed populations containing a higher percentage of patients infected with HCV.
  - A phase III study of doxorubicin versus nolatrexed was conducted in a mainly Western population in which the percentage of patients with HBV was greater in the nolatrexed than doxorubicin arm (26% vs. 18%, respectively) and vice versa for patients with HCV (36% on nolatrexed vs. 43% on doxorubicin). Although the progression-free survival times were similar, overall survival was superior with doxorubicin than nolatrexed (32.3 vs. 22.3 weeks, respectively; hazard ratio = 0.753; $P = 0.0068$).[36]
  - In contrast, a randomized phase II study of doxorubicin versus nolatrexed conducted in a Chinese population, 78% of whom were infected with HBV, showed a nonsignificant survival trend favoring nolatrexed over doxorubicin (20 vs. 15 weeks, respectively; $P = 0.98$).[37]
- The applicability of different staging and prognostic scoring systems must take into account the populations from

which they were developed. For example, the Chinese University Prognostic Index (CUPI) was derived from an all ethnic Chinese patient population seen at a single institution in Hong Kong, the majority of whom had HBV.[38] When the prognostic power of the Cancer of the Liver Italian Program (CLIP) score was evaluated in a goodness-of-fit test in the CUPI population, it performed poorly. It should be noted that the CLIP score was derived in a European patient population, 86% of whom were infected with HCV.[39] It appears that ethno-geographic factors interact with disease biology and must be considered.

- These observations represent the first steps toward a future in which HCC will likely be classified by an etiology-based genetic signature that is treated with therapies tailored to that signature.

■ References

1. Kaposi-Novak P, Lee JS, Gomez-Quiroz L, et al. Met-regulated expression signature defines a subset of human hepatocellular carcinomas with poor prognosis and aggressive phenotype. *J Clin Invest* 2006;116:1582–1595.
2. Villanueva A, Chiang DY, Newell P, et al. Pivotal role of mTOR signaling in hepatocellular carcinoma. *Gastroenterology* 2008;135:1972–1983.
3. Baba H, Wohlschlaeger J, Cicinnati VR, et al. Phosphorylation of p70S6 kinase predicts survival in patients with clear-margin resected hepatocellular carcinoma. *Liver Int* 2009 29: 399–405.
4. Hayashi H, Sugio K, Matsumata T, et al. The clinical significance of p53 gene mutation in hepatocellular carcinomas from Japan. *Hepatology* 1995;22:1702–1707.
5. Honda K, Sbisa E, Tullo A, et al. P53 mutation is a poor prognostic indicator for survival in patients with hepatocellular carcinoma undergoing surgical tumour ablation. *Br J Cancer* 1998;77:776–782.
6. Imbeaud S, Ladeiro Y, Zucman-Rossi J. Identification of novel oncogenes and tumor suppressors in hepatocellular carcinoma. *Semin Liver Dis* 2001;30:75–86.
7. Ji J, Wang XW. New kids on the block: diagnostic and prognostic microRNAs in hepatocellular carcinoma. *Cancer Biol Ther* 2009;8:1686–1693.
8. Bolondi L, Caspary W, Bennouna J, et al. Clinical benefit of sorafenib in hepatitis C patients with hepatocellular

carcinoma (HCC): subgroup analysis of the SHARP trial. 2008 Gastrointestinal Cancers Symposium, January 19–21, 2008, Orlando, FL, Abstract 129.

9.   Giambartolomei S, Covone F, Levrero M, et al. Sustained activation of the Raf/MEK/Erk pathway in response to EGF in stable cell lines expressing the hepatitis C virus (HCV) core protein. *Oncogene* 2001;20:2606–2610.

10. Huitzil FD, Saltz LS, Song J, et al. Retrospective analysis of outcome in hepatocellular carcinoma (HCC) patients (pts) with hepatitis C (C+) versus B (B+) treated with sorafenib (S). 2008 Gastrointestinal Cancers Symposium, January 19–21, 2008, Orlando, FL, Abstract 173.

11. Mejias M, Garcia-Pras E, Tiani C, et al. Beneficial effects of sorafenib on splanchnic, intrahepatic, and portocollateral circulations in portal hypertensive and cirrhotic rats. *Hepatology* 2009;49:1245–1256.

12. Abou-Alfa GK. Education session: even patients with liver dysfunction can get chemotherapy! Liver dysfunction studies. Gastrointestinal (noncolorectal) Cancer Track. 2010 American Society of Clinical Oncology Annual Meeting, June 4–8, 2010, Chicago, IL.

13. Miller AA, Murry DJ, Owzar K, et al. Phase I and pharmacokinetic study of sorafenib in patients with hepatic or renal dysfunction: CALGB 60301. *J Clin Oncol* 2009;27:1800–1805.

14. Pinter M, Sieghart W, Graziadei I, et al. Sorafenib in unresectable hepatocellular carcinoma from mild to advanced stage liver cirrhosis. *Oncologist* 2009;14:70–76.

15. Yau T, Chan P, Ng K, et al. Efficacy and tolerability of single agent sorafenib in poor risk advanced hepatocellular carcinoma patients [abstract]. *J Clin Oncol* 2008;26(Suppl):15513.

16. Abou-Alfa GK, Amadori D, Santoro A, et al. Is sorafenib (S) safe and effective in patients (pts) with hepatocellular carcinoma (HCC) and Child-Pugh B (CPB) cirrhosis? *J Clin Oncol* 2008;26(Suppl):217s.

17. Abou-Alfa GK, Schwartz L, Ricci S, et al. Phase II study of sorafenib in patients with advanced hepatocellular carcinoma. *J Clin Oncol* 2006;24:1–8.

18. Toh H, Chen P, Carr BI, et al. Linifanib phase II trial in patients with advanced hepatocellular carcinoma (HCC) [abstract]. *J Clin Oncol* 2010;28(Suppl 15s):4038.

19. Rosenberg WM, Voelker M, Thiel R, et al. Serum markers detect the presence of liver fibrosis: a cohort study. *Gastroenterology* 2004;127:1704–1713.

20. Cheng AL, Kang YK, Chen Z, et al. Efficacy and safety of sorafenib in patients in the Asia-Pacific region with advanced hepatocellular carcinoma: a phase III randomised, double-blind, placebo-controlled trial. *Lancet Oncol* 2009; 10:25–34.

21. Llovet JM, Ricci S, Mazzaferro V, et al; SHARP Investigators Study Group. Sorafenib in advanced hepatocellular carcinoma. *N Engl J Med* 2008;359:378–390.
22. Abou-Alfa GK, Zhao B, Capanu M, et al. Tumor necrosis as a correlate for response in subgroup of patients with advanced hepatocellular carcinoma (HCC) treated with sorafenib. ESMO 2008, Stockholm, Sweden, Abstract 547P.
23. Siegel AB, Cohen EI, Ocean A, et al. Phase II trial evaluating the clinical and biologic effects of bevacizumab in unresectable hepatocellular carcinoma. *J Clin Oncol* 2008;26:2992–2998.
24. Abou-Alfa GK, Gultekin DH, Capanu M, et al. Association of dynamic contrast enhanced-MRI (DCE-MRI) with response in a subgroup of patients with advanced hepatocellular carcinoma (HCC) treated with doxorubicin plus sorafenib. 2009 Gastrointestinal Cancers Symposium, San Francisco, CA, Abstract 271.
25. Jain RK, Duda DG, Clark JW, et al. Lessons from phase III clinical trials on anti-VEGF therapy for cancer. *Nat Clin Pract Oncol* 2006;3:24–40.
26. Wang FH, Yip YC, Zhang M, et al. Diagnostic utility of glypican-3 for hepatocellular carcinoma on liver needle biopsy. *J Clin Pathol* 2010;63:599–603.
27. Motomura Y, Senju S, Nakatsura T, et al. Embryonic stem cell-derived dendritic cells expressing glypican-3, a recently identified oncofetal antigen, induce protective immunity against highly metastatic mouse melanoma, B16-F10. *Cancer Res* 2006;66:2414–2422.
28. Ishiguro T, Sugimoto M, Kinoshita Y, et al. Anti-glypican 3 antibody as a potential antitumor agent for human liver cancer. *Cancer Res* 2008;68:9832–9838.
29. Sasaki Y, Yamada T, Tanaka H, et al. Risk of recurrence in a long-term follow-up after surgery in 417 patients with hepatitis B- or hepatitis C-related hepatocellular carcinoma. *Ann Surg* 2006;244:771–780.
30. Roayaie S, Haim MB, Emre S, et al. Comparison of surgical outcomes for hepatocellular carcinoma in patients with hepatitis B versus hepatitis C: a Western experience. *Ann Surg Oncol* 2000;7:764–770.
31. Huitzil FD, Saltz LS, Song J, et al. Retrospective analysis of outcome in hepatocellular carcinoma (HCC) patients (pts) with hepatitis C (C+) versus B (B+) treated with sorafenib (S). 2008 Gastrointestinal Cancers Symposium, January 19–21, 2008, Orlando, FL, Abstract 173.
32. Tiollais P, Hsu TY, Moroy T, et al. Hepadenavirus as an insertional mutagen in hepatocellular carcinoma. In: Hollinger FB, Lemon SM, Margolis HS (eds). *Viral Hepatitis and Liver Disease*. Baltimore: Williams & Wilkins, 1990:541–546.

33. Wang XW, Forrester K, Yeh H, et al. Hepatitis B virus X protein inhibits p53 sequence-specific DNA binding, transcriptional activity and association with transcription factor ERCC3. *Proc Natl Acad Sci USA* 1994;91:2230–2234.
34. Truant R, Antunovic J, Greenblatt J, et al. Direct interaction of the hepatitis B virus HBX protein with p53 leads to inhibition by HBX of p53 response element-directed transactivation. *J Virol* 1995;69:1851–1859.
35. Hayashi H, Sugio K, Matsumata T, et al. The clinical significance of p53 gene mutation in hepatocellular carcinomas from Japan. *Hepatology* 1995;22:1702–1707.
36. Gish RG, Porta C, Lazar L, et al. Phase III randomized controlled trial comparing the survival of patients with unresectable hepatocellular carcinoma treated with nolatrexed or doxorubicin. *J Clin Oncol* 2007;25:3069–3075.
37. Mok TS, Leung TW, Lee SD, et al. A multi-centre randomized phase II study of nolatrexed versus doxorubicin in treatment of Chinese patients with advanced hepatocellular carcinoma. *Cancer Chemother Pharmacol* 1999;44:307–311.
38. Leung T, Tang A, Zee B, et al. Construction of the Chinese University Prognostic Index for hepatocellular carcinoma and comparison with the TNM staging system, the Okuda staging system, and the Cancer of the Liver Italian Program staging system. A study based on 926 patients. *Cancer* 2002;94:1760–1769.
39. The Cancer of the Liver Italian Program (CLIP) Investigators. Prospective validation of the CLIP score: a new prognostic system for patients with cirrhosis and hepatocellular carcinoma. *Hepatology* 2000;31:840–845.

Index

www.ingramcontent.com/pod-product-compliance
Lightning Source LLC
Chambersburg PA
CBHW070727220326
41598CB00024BA/3337